Atlas of EEG
& Seizure Semiology

Bassel Abou-Khalil, M.D.

Professor of Neurology
& Director of the Clinical Epilepsy Program
Vanderbilt University School of Medicine
Nashville, Tennessee

Karl E Misulis M.D.,Ph.D.

Clinical Professor Neurology
Vanderbilt University School of Medicine
Nashville, Tennessee
& Neurologist, Semmes-Murphey Clinic
Jackson, Tennessee

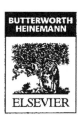

BUTTERWORTH
HEINEMANN

ELSEVIER

BUTTERWORTH
HEINEMANN

The Curtis Center
170 S Independence Mall W 300E
Philadelphia, Pennsylvania 19106

ATLAS OF EEG AND SEIZURE SEMIOLOGY

Notice
Medicine is an ever-changing field. Standard safety precautions must be followed, but as new research and clinical experience broaden our knowledge, changes in treatment and drug therapy may become necessary or appropriate. Readers are advised to check the most current product information provided by the manufacturer of each drug to be administered to verify the recommended dose, the method of duration of administration, and contraindications. It is the responsibility of the licensed prescriber, relying on experience and knowledge of the patient, to determine dosages and the best treatment for each individual patient. Neither the publisher nor the author assumes any liability for any injury and/or damage to persons or property arising from this publication.
The Publisher

Library of Congress Cataloging-in-Publication Data

Abou-Khalil, Bassel
Atlas of EEG & seizure semiology / Bassel Abou-Khalil, Karl E. Misulis
    p.   ;cm.
        Includes bibliographical references.
        ISBN-13: 978-0-7506-7513-0   ISBN-10: 0-7506-7513-6
    1. Electroencephalography--Atlases. 2. Epilepsy—Atlases. 3. Convulsions—Atlases.
        I. Title: Atlas of EEG and seizure semiology. II. Misulis, Karl E. III. Title.
        [DNLM: 1. Electroencephalography—methods—Atlases. 2. Seizures—diagnosis—Atlases. WL 17 A155a
        2006]
        RC386.6.E43A26 2006
        616.8'047547—dc22

ISBN-13: 978-0-7506-7513-0   2005050133
ISBN-10: 0-7506-7513-6

Acquisitions Editor: Susan Pioli
Developmental Editor: Laurie Anello

Printed in the United States of America
Last digit is the print number: 9 8 7 6 5 4 3

For our families.

Preface

As we go further into the present millennium, we look back on the development of medicine, and specifically neurophysiology and are amazed at the advances we have made. Undoubtedly, at the end of this century, our descendents will look on our present technology as quaint and wonder how we were able to use these tools to assist patient care.

This atlas presents a concise manual for performance and interpretation of EEG in clinical practice. The small book is an introduction to raise all readers to a basic level of understanding. The disc presents some of the same information plus extensive examples of EEG recordings from routine and video EEG monitoring, as well as video recording of seizures.

The authors chose to adhere mainly to the older and more widely used classification schemes rather than the less widely used yet thoughtful schemes that are in development. Future editions of this work will reflect new schemes when fully established.

In an effort to keep this work at a manageable size, the authors have had to be selective, and as a result have omitted or limited discussion of some clinical and electrophysiologic entities.

The information contained in this work is distilled from many years of clinical experience and thousands of scientific papers. In this concise text, it was impossible to list all of these valuable works. The authors would like to express their appreciation to all of those colleagues who provided examples and information and to all of those who have contributed to the knowledge base in this field.

The authors would also like to express their appreciation to Susan F. Pioli and her staff at Elsevier and to all of the technicians, assistants, and patients without whom this project would have been impossible.

Bassel Abou-Khalil and Karl E. Misulis

April 2005

Contents

Atlas of EEG & Seizure Semiology

Chapter 1. Introduction

Physiology

Membrane physiology

Neuronal membranes are composed of lipid bilayers, which have transmembrane proteins. These proteins form the channels through which ions have differential permeability. The sodium-potassium pump uses energy to maintain the ionic gradients, which are important for intact neuronal function. At rest, potassium is sequestered inside the cell whereas sodium is excluded from the cell. At rest, there is a greater permeability to potassium than other ions. During an action potential, there is greater permeability to sodium.

Diffusion potential

The diffusion potential is established by efflux of potassium, which travels down its chemical gradient until the resulting electrical gradient opposes further efflux of ions. The potential at which there is electrochemical equilibrium is approximately 75 mV for most neurons, with the inside negative.

The diffusion potential is essential for generation of the depolarization, which will occur with electrotonic conduction, and action potentials.

Electrotonic conduction

Depolarization of a segment of membrane results in activation of *sodium channels*. These allow the influx of sodium down its electrical and chemical gradient. The influx continues until the channel closes after a defined period of time, the *open time*. Therefore, channel opening is *voltage dependent*, i.e. dependent on the membrane potential, whereas closing of the channels is *time dependent*. After the channel is closed, it cannot be opened until a fixed period has elapsed, i.e. the refractory period.

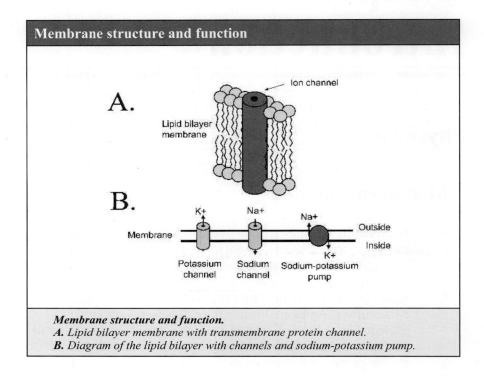

Membrane structure and function.
A. *Lipid bilayer membrane with transmembrane protein channel.*
B. *Diagram of the lipid bilayer with channels and sodium-potassium pump.*

Depolarization of one segment of membrane results in depolarization of adjacent membrane by *electrotonic conduction*. This type of conduction does not use energy, but decays along the length of the membrane. If the electrotonic depolarization of the membrane is sufficient, an action potential can develop.

Post-synaptic potentials

Post-synaptic potentials are created by the release of neurotransmitter onto the post-synaptic membrane. Excitatory transmitters such as acetylcholine and glutamate produce depolarization by opening of sodium and/or calcium channels. The depolarization can be recorded intracellularly as an *excitatory post-synaptic potential* (EPSP).

Inhibitory transmitters such as GABA produce opening of potassium and/or chloride channels, which results in loss of excitability not so much by hyperpolarization of the membrane, but rather by clamping of the membrane potential near the equilibrium potential for these ions, which is far from threshold. For example, the depolarization that would normally be produced by opening of sodium channels is blunted by the action of inhibitory transmitters essentially locking the membrane potential near the equilibrium potential for potassium. The potential produced is the *inhibitory post-synaptic potential* (IPSP).

Action potential

The action potential is due to regenerative opening of sodium channels. The channel opening results in depolarization of adjacent membrane which then causes sodium channels in these areas to open, thereby perpetuating the depolarization. The channels close in a time-dependent fashion.

Therefore, channel opening is *voltage dependent*, whereas the closing is *time dependent*. There is a brief *refractory period* before the channel can be opened again to create the next action potential.

Generators of EEG potentials

EEG activity is due to charge movement in neuronal membranes. It is attractive to think of EEG activity as originating in defined nuclei, but in general, the electrical potentials represent the summed electrical activity from a substantial number of neurons.

EEG recorded from the scalp is generated by the cerebral cortex, with the portion of the cortex adjacent to the skull being the largest contributor.

Cortical potentials

Most cortical efferents are oriented perpendicular to the cortical surface. The gyration of the cortex results in only a fraction of the cortical efferents being oriented perpendicular to the scalp. Therefore, those pyramidal neurons that are oriented perpendicular to the scalp would be expected to have a disparate contribution to the surface-recorded EEG. Electrical activity at the large cortical pyramidal neurons produces dipoles which are summed to generate the scalp EEG.

It is thought that summated EPSPs and IPSPs are responsible for most of the EEG activity recorded at the scalp. Surprisingly, action potentials probably have a minimal contribution to the EEG. The longer duration of postsynaptic potentials is more in line with the duration of most scalp recorded EEG activity, whereas action potentials are too short.

Scalp potentials

Scalp electrodes are unable to see all of the electrical activity of the brain. Synchronous activity of numerous neurons is required for there to be a recordable wave from the scalp leads. One estimate is that approximately 6 cm^2 of cortical surface must be synchronously activated in order for there to be a potential recorded at the surface. Scalp potentials are volume conducted through the skull and scalp, which results in considerable attenuation of the activity. There is greater attenuation of potentials that rise and fall rapidly, i.e. higher frequency potentials.

Generation of abnormal EEG activity

The most important types of abnormal EEG activity are attenuation, slow activity, and epileptiform activity. Attenuation indicates desynchronization or reduction of electrocerebral activity. Slowing indicates disordered function of the neurons. Epileptiform activity indicates abnormal synchronous activity.

Attenuation

Focal attenuation

Focal attenuation usually indicates a cortical lesion or reversible cortical dysfunction, since EEG activity is generated at the cortex. Focal attenuation could also result from an increase in tissue between the cortex and the recording electrode.

Since each EEG channel displays the potential difference between electrodes, attenuation will be seen if there is reduction in potential difference between electrodes in a channel. In bipolar recordings where each channel displays the difference between adjacent electrodes, attenuation will be seen if there is an electrical shunt eliminating the potential difference. Such a shunt can be due to smeared conductive electrode gel connecting the two electrodes, or a chronic subdural hematoma.

Generalized attenuation

Generalized attenuation may suggest a generalized cortical injury or transient dysfunction. However, an attenuated EEG in adults could be a normal variant.

Slow activity

Focal slow activity

Focal irregular slow activity is usually due to a localized subcortical structural lesion (or dysfunction). Focal slow activity seems to be a result of deafferentation of the cortex from subcortical structures.

Generalized bisynchronous slow activity

Generalized bisynchronous slow activity can be intermittent or continuous. It is felt to be due to disordered circuit loops between cortex and thalamus. This type of abnormality is reported in conditions affecting both cortical and subcortical structures, as well as in a number of toxic/metabolic encephalopathies, and in deep midline lesions. In the latter situation, generalized bisynchronous slow activity may be referred to as a projected rhythm.

Generalized asynchronous slow activity

Generalized asynchronous slow activity has a broad differential diagnosis, though it usually indicates encephalopathy. Some of the possibilities include degenerative processes, encephalitis, extensive multifocal vascular disease, and toxic and metabolic disorders.

Epileptiform activity

Epileptiform activity involves abnormal synchronous activation of many neurons. Corresponding to focal epileptiform activity at the cellular level is a wave of depolarization called the *paroxysmal depolarization shift* (PDS).

Paroxysmal depolarization shift

The PDS is the fundamental electrophysiological substrate of focal epileptiform activity. The PDS cannot be recorded with scalp electrodes but requires cortical microelectrodes for detection.

Paroxysmal depolarization shift

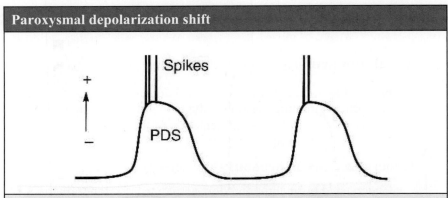

The PDS is a prolonged phase of depolarization, which can be sufficient to produce multiple action potentials. For this illustration the duration is brief and the discharge would be interictal, but markedly prolonged PDS are possible and can be associated with an ictal discharge.

The PDS is an extracellular field potential where there is a wave of depolarization followed by a wave of repolarization. High-amplitude afferent input to the cortex produces depolarization of cortical neurons sufficient to trigger repetitive action potentials, which in turn contribute to the potentials recorded at the surface. Repolarization due to inactivation of interneurons is followed by a brief period of hyperpolarization.

Cyclic depolarization and repolarization is believed to be the cortical counterpart to rhythmic spike-and-wave discharges seen sometimes in epilepsy. The rhythmicity may be at least in part due to the inability of cortical neurons to sustain prolonged high frequency discharges but in addition is likely due to built-in circuitry to inhibit repetitive discharges. The repetitive discharge is not terminated by neuronal exhaustion but rather by this mechanism of inactivation. Recent data suggest that there may be membrane effects independent of active inhibition to terminate seizures, yet the exact mechanisms of seizure termination are still under study.

Spikes and sharp waves

Sustained depolarization of a neuron can result in multiple action potentials on the crest of the depolarization. If one neuron is activated by this burst, there will likely be no neurologic symptoms and the discharge will not be recorded from scalp electrodes. However, if there is synchronous activation of multiple neurons, this can be recorded on scalp electrodes as a spike or sharp wave.

Spikes and sharp waves generated at the crown of a gyrus have a radial (perpendicular, vertical) dipole, with surface negativity. The positive end of the dipole is subcortical, and can be recorded only with a depth electrode. If discharges are generated totally or partially within a fissure, the dipole may be tangent (parallel, horizontal). One remarkable example is in rolandic epilepsy, where the positive end of the dipole is often in the frontal region, and is visible on routine recording in most of these patients.

Dipole

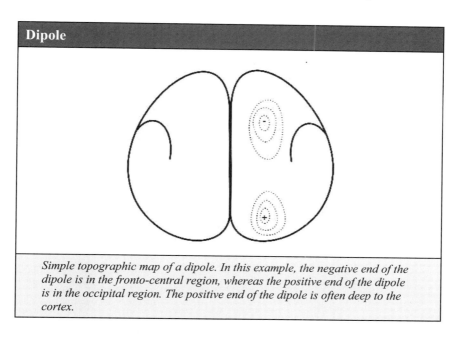

Simple topographic map of a dipole. In this example, the negative end of the dipole is in the fronto-central region, whereas the positive end of the dipole is in the occipital region. The positive end of the dipole is often deep to the cortex.

Spikes and sharp waves are occasionally surface positive. In neonates positive spikes and sharp waves may have a particular significance due to association with intraventricular hemorrhage.

Seizure

There is a grey zone between interictal activity and ictal activity. Repetitive discharge on the crest of the PDS may be prolonged to produce a seizure. In addition, a prolonged discharge of one neuron may then entrain a group of adjacent neurons to depolarize and repetitively discharge, thereby producing expansion of the region of epileptogenic activity and prolongation of the discharge to clear ictal duration.

Chapter 2.
EEG Technology

Electrodes

Electrode basics

Electrodes are connected to the scalp with a conducting gel, which serves a malleable extension of the electrode. Without this extension, any minor movement of the head would result in mechanical disturbance of the electrode-scalp interface, producing electrical artifact.

For most purposes, electrode basics are unimportant to day-to-day performance of EEG. Details of electrode function are discussed on the disc and in *Essentials of Clinical Neurophysiology* (Misulis and Head, Elsevier, 2003).

Some important technical requirements of electrodes and electrode placement are as follows:

- Electrodes of the same type and manufacturer
- Equal lead length
- Equal electrode impedances
- Leads are not in proximity to other devices
- Leads are not coiled

Electrodes should all be of good condition and be of the same type and manufacturer.

Electrode placement

Electrodes are usually placed according the *10-20 System*. This is a widely accepted method of electrode lead placement, which takes advantage of measurement of the skull with defined landmarks. Details of the electrode placement system are presented on the disc. A diagram of the electrode placements is shown in the figure.

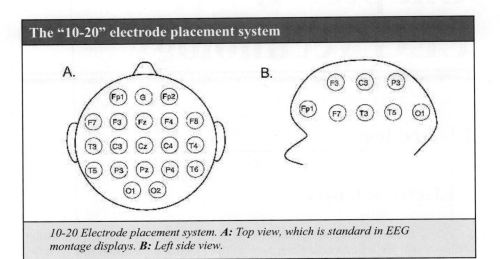

The "10-20" electrode placement system

*10-20 Electrode placement system. **A:** Top view, which is standard in EEG montage displays. **B:** Left side view.*

Terminology for scalp electrodes is such that

- Each electrode has a two or three character component, letters and numbers. The first character(s) indicate the general cerebral region, and the last character indicates the area in that region.
- The regions for the first character are frontopolar (Fp), frontal (F), central (C), temporal (T), parietal (P), occipital (O).
- For the second character, odd numbers are left hemisphere, even numbers are right hemisphere, and the lower-case "z" is midline.

Therefore, C3 is in the left central region approximately overlying the rolandic region. C4 is over the corresponding area on the right hemisphere.

Full names for electrodes

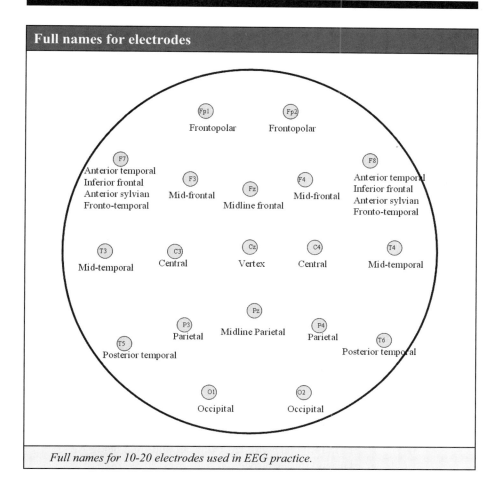

Full names for 10-20 electrodes used in EEG practice.

Notice that F7 and F8 have several names, reflecting that they can record both anterior temporal or inferior frontal activity. Examining the field of discharges may be essential to determine the source of recorded activity. For example, if the field is F8 and T4, then F8 activity is anterior temporal, while if the field is F4 and F8, then F8 is likely recording inferior frontal activity. If F8 alone is involved, or if the field involves F8 and Fp2 (Fp2 records frontopolar activity but could also detect dipoles originating at the temporal tip), then it is not clear if F8 is anterior temporal or inferior frontal, hence the name anterior sylvian (our preferred term) or frontotemporal. This uncertain status of F7/F8 has resulted in the exploration of "true" anterior temporal electrodes (see page 12).

Potential fields

Field distribution on the scalp. See text for discussion. The left field suggests that activity in an inferior frontal location whereas on the right is an anterior temporal location.

On the left the field suggests that F8 is an inferior frontal electrode, whereas on the right the field suggests that it is an anterior temporal electrode.

Other leads of interest include:

- Ear (auricular) with left being A1 and right being A2
- Ground (G) electrode

Additional electrodes outside the 10-20 system

Additional leads are occasionally placed, although not as part of routine EEG performance. These include *Silverman "true" anterior temporal (T1 and T2) electrodes*, to monitor anterior temporal activity, zygomatic electrodes and cheek electrodes, for monitoring of lateral-basal temporal lobe activity, and supraorbital electrodes, for monitoring anterior orbitofrontal activity. The reason for the T1/T2 electrodes is that F7/F8, which are the anterior temporal electrodes of the 10-20 system, are physically located over the lateral inferior-posterior frontal region. They do record anterior temporal lobe activity, but may also record frontal activity. To monitor mesial-basal temporal activity, the most commonly used electrodes are sphenoidal electrodes.

Nasopharyngeal electrodes (Pg) were frequently used in the past, but are rarely used now because they are unstable, easily dislodged, and become more uncomfortable over time.

Deep sphenoidal (Sp) electrodes are inserted with a spinal needle, just below the zygomatic arch, 2 cm anterior to the line between the tragus and the condyle of the mandible. The needle is directed horizontally and approximately 10 degrees posteriorly. The tip should rest close to the foramen ovale (at a depth of 4-5 cm). Although their insertion is painful, sphenoidal electrodes are well tolerated and stable, making them ideal for recording seizures with long-term monitoring.

Mini-sphenoidal electrodes are inserted in the same location to a depth of only 1 cm. This makes them possible to insert by EEG technologists. Although they are not as good as sphenoidal electrodes for detecting mesial-basal activity, their ease of insertion makes them useful for short-term recordings.

T1 electrode placement

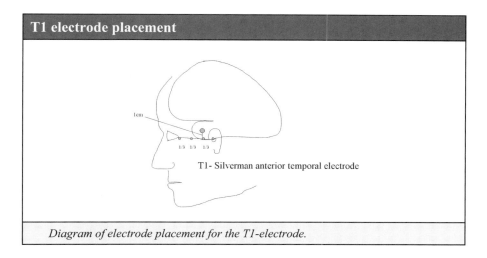

Diagram of electrode placement for the T1-electrode.

T1 electrode placement: The distance from the auditory canal to the outer canthus of the eye is measured and divided in thirds. T1 will be one cm superior to the mark closest to the ear canal.

10-10 system

The 10-10 electrode placement system is based on the same landmarks as the 10-20 system, but involves the addition of electrodes in between 10-20 electrode positions. Although there have been several nomenclatures for this system, the one recommended by the American EEG Society (now the American Clinical Neurophysiology Society), is the modified combinatorial nomenclature. In this nomenclature system, the letters identify the location, particularly the coronal plane location, and the number (or z) refers to the position relative to the midline. The odd numbers (1 to 9) belong on the left, the even numbers (2 to 10) belong on the right, and z still stands for the midline. The smaller numbers refer to positions close to the midline and the larger numbers to positions further away from the midline. In this new nomenclature, the 10-20 electrode names could be preserved, with the exception of T3/T4 and T5/T6. These electrodes lie in the same sagittal planes as F7 and F8 and needed to have the same numbers. T3 and T4 were therefore changed to T7 and T8. T5 and T6, the posterior temporal electrodes are close to the temporo-parieto-occipital junction, and as they are in the same coronal plane as P3 and P4, were named P7 and P8. In this atlas, both new and old names for these electrodes are used.

The additional coronal electrodes planes created in the 10-10 system are AF for anterior frontal, FC and FT for frontocentral and frontotemporal plane, CP and TP for centroparietal and temporoparietal plane, and PO for parieto-occipital plane. Additional electrodes in the 10-10 system are rarely used in routine EEG recording. Even in epilepsy monitoring it would be very impractical to use all the 10-10 electrodes. However, when the field of certain activity has to be clarified, selected additional electrodes can be used in a region of interest. For example in suspected mesial frontocentral foci, FC1, FCz, FC2, C1, C2, CP1, CPz, and CP2 could be added for best delineation of the field. In left temporal lobe epilepsy, FT7, FT9, and T9 could be added and may obviate the need for T1 and T2 electrodes.

Electrode positions of the 10-20 system

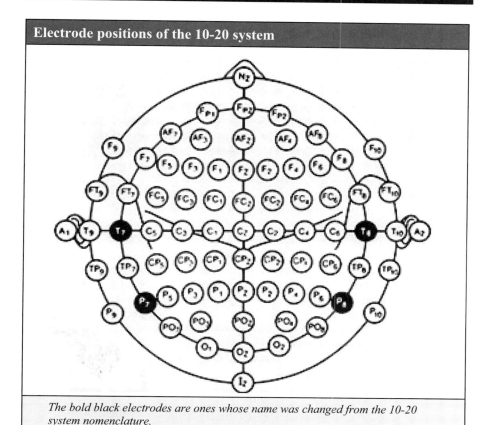

The bold black electrodes are ones whose name was changed from the 10-20 system nomenclature.

The following are the new and old names for the revised 10-20 system

- T7 = T3
- T8 = T4
- P7 = T5
- P8 = T6

Physiologic monitoring

It is often important to monitor physiological parameter in conjunction with the EEG. EKG is the most important and needs to be monitored in all patients. One reason is that EKG artifact often appears on EEGs and could result in confusion regarding the origin of some sharp potentials. Additional electrodes for physiological monitoring need to be used predominantly in neonatal EEGs, in brain death recordings, and in select situations, particularly for ICU recordings.

Additional electrodes include, but are not restricted to the following:

- Eye movement electrodes
  - o Infraorbital electrodes (these are placed immediately below each eye, for distinguishing vertical eye movements from frontal EEG activity)
  - o Electro-oculogram leads (both electrodes are lateral to the eyes, one above the right eye, and another electrode below the left eye). These leads record eye movements. They are used mainly for neonatal EEG and for sleep recordings
- Submental EMG electrodes
- Respiration monitor (to monitor respiratory effort)
- Air flow monitor

EEG technologists should be encouraged to be proactive and creative adding electrodes as needed. For example, if the patient has right arm jerks and EEG potentials that may be linked to these, the tech could add an electrode over the right arm, that would help the electroencephalographer in identifying a consistent relationship between the jerk artifact and the EEG potentials.

Electrode application

There are two basic ways to attach electrodes to the scalp, gel and collodion. Gel is used mainly for office and hospital short-term studies. Collodion is used when stability of the electrodes is especially important, such as for long-term monitoring and ambulatory patients.

Electrode application using gel is as follows:

- Locate the positions for electrodes using the 10-20 Electrode Placement System
- Separate strands of hair over the electrode positions using the wooden end of a cotton-tipped applicator
- Clean dead skin and dirt from the region with a mildly abrasive cleaning agent such as Omni-Prep or NuPrep using the cotton-tipped applicator
- Scoop some electrode paste into the electrode
- Place the electrode in position over the skin
- Put a 2"x2" gauze pad over the electrode and push it firmly onto the head, providing a seal that prevents the electrode from falling off the scalp

Application of electrodes with collodion involves the following steps:

- Prepare the head at the electrode positions as mentioned above.
- Place the electrode on the scalp
- Place a piece of gauze soaked with collodion over the electrode
- Use compressed air to dry the collodion
- Insert a blunt-tipped needle into the cup and scrape the skin to lower electrode impedance
- Inject electrolyte (electrode gel) into the cup of the electrode using the blunt-tipped needle.

Removal of paste-fixed electrodes is easy. The gauze pads are pulled off then the electrodes gently pulled off, tilting them to release the vacuum effect that holds them on. Then, the paste left on the scalp can be largely removed by rubbing with a warm, wet wash cloth. After the patient washes the hair that evening, all traces of the recording are gone.

Removal of collodion-fixed electrodes is more difficult. First, the collodion is softened by use of acetone, then the areas cleaned as above. The degree of washing required is greater both immediately by the technician and later by the patient. Some patients object to the acetone smell more than any other part of the procedure.

Each method has its advantages. Collodion provides a more secure attachment and is more suitable for long-term recordings. Electrode paste is easier to apply and remove and is suitable for most routine office and hospital recordings.

Routine EEG

EEG is performed in a variety of montages, so EEG can be assessed with a spectrum of presentations. For example, a spike may be more visible on one montage than another. Modern digital machines have the ability to change montage while displaying the same epoch, adding extra interpretive flexibility.

Rules of polarity

All EEG channels have two inputs. Each EEG channel represents the difference in potential between two adjacent electrodes. In referential montages (see below), the active electrode is in the first input and a presumably neutral reference is in the second input. Because of that the first input has been called "active" input and second input "reference" input. However, in bipolar montages (and in the instance of an active reference), the active electrode can be in either the first or second input. By convention, a negative potential in the first input is seen as an upward deflection, whereas a positive potential in the first input is seen as downward deflection. Potentials arising in the second input will have the reverse appearance.

Table: Polarity convention		
EEG activity	*Input 1*	*Input 2*
Negative	Up	Down
Positive	Down	Up

The term "active" and "reference" are really misnomers. For bipolar montages adjacent electrodes are usually connected in the two inputs. By convention, the more anterior electrode or the left-sided electrode is connected to the active input, and the more posterior electrode or right-sided electrode is connected to the second or reference input. The "reference" input can be just as active as the "active" input - positive 10 mV at the "reference" electrode will give the same deflection of the pen or computer display as negative 10 mV at the "active" electrode. The recording is an arithmetic subtraction between the "active" and "reference" electrode potentials. In the remainder of this book, we will use the terminology of *input 1* or *first input* and *input 2* or *second input*.

Montages

Montages are created so that viewing the EEG gives the neurophysiologist a clear picture of the spatial distribution of EEG across the cortex. Because of this, many neurophysiologists have their favorite montages, though they realize they should view multiple montages in a recording. A good montage is one that can be easily imagined and remembered. It should also have equal electrode distances within each chain (unless it includes electrodes outside the 10-20 system, such as sphenoidal electrodes).

Montages

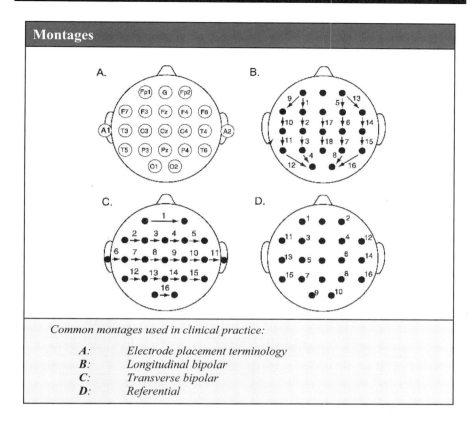

Common montages used in clinical practice:

A: Electrode placement terminology
B: Longitudinal bipolar
C: Transverse bipolar
D: Referential

Montage guidelines

The *American Electroencephalographic Society Guidelines in EEG, Evoked Potentials, and Polysomnography* (1994) have made basic recommendations for montages as well as other technical aspects of performing routine EEG. These will be called the *Guidelines*, for the rest of this text.

The guidelines recommend the following:

- Record at least 8 channels
- Use the full 21-electrode array of the 10-20 System
- Every routine recording session should include at least one montage from each of the following groups: referential, longitudinal bipolar, and transverse bipolar
- Label each montage in the recording
- Use simple montages that allow for easy visualization of the spatial orientation of the waveforms - for example, bipolar montages should be in straight lines with equal inter-electrode distances
- Have the anterior and left-sided channels above the posterior and right-sided channels

- Use at least some montages that are commonly used in other laboratories.

Most Laboratories now use digital EEG machines and are no longer restricted in the number of channels (up to 32 are allowed by most digital machines). It is therefore recommended that montages include all the midline electrodes as well as EKG.

Recommended montages for routine use in adults and children after the neonatal period are shown in the table below. Additional channels are used when available and needed. The additional channels may be used for ECG, eye movements, respirations, or EMG.

Table: Montages

Channel	Longitudinal bipolar (LB)	Transverse bipolar (TB)	Average reference (Ave)	Ipsilateral ear reference (Ipsi)*	Circum-ferential (CIR)
1	Fp1 – F3	F7 – Fp1	Fp1 – Ave	Fp1 – A1	T3 – F7
2	F3 – C3	Fp1 – Fp2	Fp2 – Ave	Fp2 – A2	F7 – Fp1
3	C3 – P3	Fp2 – F8	F3 – Ave	F3 – A1	Fp1 – Fp2
4	P3 – O1	F7 – F3	F4 – Ave	F4 – A2	Fp2 – F8
5	Fp2 – F4	F3 – Fz	C3 – Ave	C3 – A1	F8 – T4
6	F4 – C4	Fz – F4	C4 – Ave	C4 – A2	T3 – T5
7	C4 – P4	F4 – F8	P3 – Ave	P3 – A1	T5 – O1
8	P4 – O2	A1 – T3	P4 – Ave	P4 – A2	O1 – O2
9	Fp1 – F7	T3 – C3	O1 – Ave	O1 – A1	O2 – T6
10	F7 – T3	C3 – Cz	O2 – Ave	O2 – A2	T6 – T4
11	T3 – T5	Cz – C4	F7 – Ave	F7 – A1	Fp1 – F3
12	T5 – O1	C4 – T4	F8 – Ave	F8 – A2	F3 – C3
13	Fp2 – F8	T4 – A2	T3 – Ave	T3 – A1	C3 – O1
14	F8 – T4	T5 – P3	T4 – Ave	T4 – A2	Fp2 – F4
15	T4 – T6	P3 – Pz	T5 – Ave	T5 – A1	F4 – C4
16	T6 – O2	Pz – P4	T6 – Ave	T6 – A2	C4 – O2
17	Fz – Cz	P4 – T6	Fz – Ave	Fz – A1	Fz – Cz
18	Cz – Pz	T5 – O1	Cz – Ave	Cz – A1	Cz – Pz
19	EKG	O1 – O2	Pz- Ave	Pz – A1	EKG
20		O2 – T6	EKG	EKG	
21		EKG			

The ipsilateral ear reference (Ipsi) can be replaced with the linked reference (LE) if there is prominent EKG artifact from one or both ear references. The EKG artifact tends to be of opposite polarity on the two sides, and linking the ears will usually attenuate it or eliminate it.

More details on montages and localization are presented in the following chapter.

Recording parameters

Filters

Standard low-frequency filter (LFF) setting for routine EEG is 1 Hz. This corresponds to a time constant (TC) of 0.16 sec. If the LFF is set higher, there is distortion and attenuation of some slow waves. The waves can have an increased number of phases and seem composed of faster frequencies. The technicians should be discouraged from turning up the LFF when there is an abundance of slow activity. The low frequency filter setting can be adjusted downwards to improve the identification of suspected slow activity.

Standard high-frequency filter (HFF) setting for routine EEG is 70 Hz. This is slightly higher than line power frequency. Therefore, turning the HFF to a lower frequency will attenuate electrical artifact; however, this should be discouraged, because this will also attenuate physiological sharp activity. Changing recording situation and use of the 60-Hz filter are preferable, but still not without distortion effects.

The 60-Hertz or "Notch" filter attenuates specifically line power, 60-Hz in the US and Canada and 50-Hz in the UK. The 60-Hz filter is not needed in most patients in office practice, because the office laboratories are electrically protected. However, in a hospital or especially ICU setting, the filter may be required in order for line artifact to not obscure the recording. The filter should not be used to correct focal 60 Hz artifact, which is most likely related to focally increased electrode impedance. Focal 60 Hz artifact should prompt the technologist to perform an electrode impedance check and correct electrode impedances.

Digital filters accomplish the same tasks as analog filters, and are essentially calculations performed on the arrays of data.

Amplifier sensitivity

Amplifier sensitivity is initially set to 7 μV/mm. Increased sensitivity is used with low-voltage recordings, most common in elderly patients in the awake state, and in pathological states of electrocerebral suppression. The sensitivity is increased to 2 μV/mm for brain death studies. Reduced sensitivity is used for patients with high-voltage EEGs, such as in children, especially in the sleeping state, and when there are high amplitude transients such as seizure discharges.

Care must be exercised when changing amplifier sensitivity with seizures. A reduction in sensitivity allows for better visualization of the discharge, but on the other hand, the EEG after the discharge may appear suppressed when there is merely a change in the display character. Digital recording allows for playback with and without sensitivity change, avoiding this potential problem.

Electrode impedance

Electrode impedance should be at least 100 ohms and no more than 5 kohms. Usually, the impedance is on the higher end of this range. Excessively high impedance indicates that there is a problem with the leads or fixation of the leads to the scalp. High electrode impedance increases noise in a couple of ways. Excessively low impedance usually indicates smear between the electrodes, and would impair visualization of electrocerebral potentials. When two electrodes are electrically connected by conductive gel/paste they act as a single large electrode. Even in referential recordings they are a problem, limiting the sharpness of localization.

Paper speed

The concept of paper speed applies not only to hard-copy EEG recordings, but also to the display of digital EEG. Typical EEG paper display is at 30 mm/sec, with slower speeds used mainly for sleep studies. Faster paper speeds are rarely used, but can help to identify small differences in the timing of epileptiform discharges in different brain regions. This can help localization of the focus. A slower paper speed (or compression of the time axis) may help in identifying low voltage low frequency activity.

Recording procedures

Modern laboratories use digital or analog EEG machines, although the digital machines will become more standard in future years. Therefore, discussions must cover both types of recording systems.

Identification of the record

Regardless of the recording type, the recording should contain the following information:

- Name
- Age
- Identification number of the patient
- Index number of the recording
- Time and date of the recording
- Clinical reason for the study
- Time of the last seizure, if appropriate
- Ordering clinician
- Current medications
- Sedative medications used
- Name of the technician
- Technical summary, including activation methods and artifacts
- Technician's observations including regions of particular interest

For analog recordings, this information is attached to the physical EEG recording. For digital recordings, this information is included with the digitized EEG data, and should be on the printed report.

Calibration

The recording begins with two phases of calibration: square-wave and biological.

Square-wave calibration: A square-wave pulse is delivered from a waveform generator into each amplifier input. This pulse is 50µV in amplitude and alternated on and off at 1 second intervals. The wave does not appear precisely square because of the effects of the preset default filters. A sample recording is shown in the figure on page 24.

Square-wave calibration

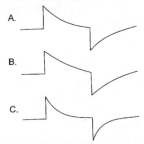

A.

B.

C.

*This is a response of the EEG amplifier equipment to different filter settings. Normal settings of HFF and LFF result in **A**. A square-wave pulse produces a quick upstroke that is followed by a slow decay to baseline. This decay occurs because this is not a DC amplifier. If the LFF is set lower, the rate of decay of the peak potential is lower as in **B**. If the LFF is set to a higher frequency, the rate of decay is faster, as in **C**.*

Biocal

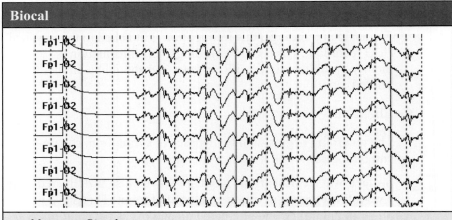

Montage = Biocal

Biocal is biological calibration of the EEG machine. Only 8 channels are shown, but all channels would be tested with identical inputs.

The low-frequency filter transforms the plateau of the signal pulse into an exponential decay. The rapidity of the decay depends on the filter setting. The lower-frequency the setting, the slower the decay. Higher settings of the LFF cause the decay to baseline to occur rapidly.

The high-frequency filter rounds off the top of the peak of the calibration. Lower settings of the HFF cause the peak to be blunted and of lower amplitude. Higher settings of the HFF cause the peak to be sharper and of higher amplitude.

We recommend trying different filter settings while recording square-wave calibration. The experienced neurophysiologist can determine an error in response of the system by abnormalities in the square-wave calibration. Some of these abnormalities include:

- Peak too rounded
- Peak overshoot
- Incorrect rate of decay
- Too low or too high amplitude of the signal

These determinations are made in comparison with other recordings and in comparison to the recordings from the other channels.

Biological calibration: Biological calibration assesses response of the amplifiers and filters to a complex biological signal, composed of a host of frequencies. A single bipolar electrode combination is fed into the active and reference electrodes of each channel. The response of each channel is seen on the Biocal pages. The recording from each channel should be identical.

Types of abnormalities of Biocal seen in one or more channels in comparison to the other channels include:

- Different amplitude
- Different frequency composition
- Improperly distributed baseline

Recording the EEG

Initial settings: The recording begins with the patient usually in the awake state with standard sensitivities and filter settings.

Electrode impedance is tested and should be at least 100 ohms and no more than 5,000 ohms.

- Initial sensitivity is set to 7 μV/mm
- High-frequency filter is set to 70 Hz
- Low-frequency filter is set to 1 Hz.

The settings may have to be changed depending on the appearance of the recording. A low-voltage record will prompt the technician to increase the sensitivity. A high-voltage record, such as is seen in some children, may require lower sensitivity. An electrically noisy recording may require activation of the 60-Hz filter. Change in HFF and LFF settings for the purpose of eliminating noise should be avoided, if at all possible.

State change: The response to state changes are recorded, since the activity may differ substantially between states. Some epileptiform activity is only present in the sleeping state. On the other hand, encephalopathy is almost impossible to diagnose when only a drowsy or sleep recording is obtained. Focal slow activity may be evident in the awake state, but disappear in the generalized slow activity of sleep. Sleep induced by sedative or sleep deprivation is a state change, but since it is induced, it is considered an activation method.

Activation methods: Photic stimulation is performed on almost all patients, although mobile equipment may not allow for photic stimulation on a portable study. Hyperventilation is performed especially when the clinical question is primary generalized epilepsy, but is generally performed on all patients who are old enough to understand the task. Hyperventilation is not performed in elderly patients or in those with advanced cardiac or cerebrovascular disease, because there is the possibility of reduction in cerebral perfusion.

Video monitoring

Montages

The montages used for video monitoring are essentially the same as those used for routine EEG. Seizures detected in an epilepsy laboratory often have a frontal or temporal origin, so particular attention is paid to those portions of the montage. Special electrodes including sphenoidal leads can be placed. Nasopharyngeal electrodes are not commonly used. When electrodes from outside the 10-20 system are used, they are usually evaluated with a referential montage, because it would be hard to include them in a bipolar montage, while still having equal inter-electrode distances. The sphenoidal electrodes are an exception to this rule. The table on page 27 shows three different bipolar and one referential montage that include sphenoidal electrodes.

Channel	Coronal Sp bipolar	LB sphenoidal	Circumferential sphenoidal	Average referential montage
1	Cz – C3	Fp1 – F3	O1 – P7	Fp1 – Ave
2	C3 – T7	F3 – C3	P7 – T7	Fp2 – Ave
3	T7 – Sp1	C3 – P3	T7 – F7	F3 – Ave
4	Sp1 – Sp2	P3 – O1	F7 – Sp1	F4 – Ave
5	Sp2 – T8	Fp2 – F4	Sp1 – Sp2	C3 – Ave
6	T8 – C4	F4 – C4	Sp2 – F8	C4 – Ave
7	C4 - Cz	C4 – P4	F8 – T8	P3 – Ave
8	Fp1 – F7	P4 – O2	T8 – P8	P4 – Ave
9	F7 – T3	Fp1 – F7	P8 – O2	O1 – Ave
10	T3 – T5	F7 – Sp1	Fp1 – F3	O2 – Ave
11	T5 – O1	Sp1 – T7	F3 – C3	F7 – Ave
12	Fp2 – F8	T7 – P7	C3 – P3	F8 – Ave
13	F8 – T4	P7 – O1	Fp2 – F4	Sp1 – Ave
14	T4 – T6	Fp2 – F8	F4 – C4	Sp2 – Ave
15	T6 – O2	F8 – Sp2	C4 – P4	T7 – Ave
16	Fz – Cz	Sp2 – T8	Fz - Cz	T8 – Ave
17	Cz – Pz	T8 – P8	Cz - Pz	P7 – Ave
18	EKG	P8 – O2	Sp1 - Pz	P8 – Ave
19		Fz – Cz	Sp2 - Pz	Fz – Ave
20		Cz – Pz	EKG	Cz – Ave
21		EKG		Pz- Ave
22				EKG

Montages for sphenoidal electrodes. The new nomenclature is used for T3/T4 (T7/T8) and T5/T6 (P7/P8). The first montage is the most commonly used, but it does not include parasagittal chains. Parasagittal chains can be added with digital recordings. The third montage is the one that the authors prefer, because it allows comparison of all temporal electrodes in one chain, including sphenoidal electrodes to each other. The referential sphenoidal channels at the bottom also help in direct comparisons of the two sphenoidal electrodes.

Recording procedures

The patient spends the entire recording epoch in the monitoring room, usually a hospital room that is especially modified and equipped for monitoring. Video recording by one or two cameras mounted high on the wall or the ceiling is recorded along with the EEG activity. The data are stored either on tape or digitally, with most modern equipment using digital video and EEG recording. Videotape recording is much less technically demanding, although more difficult to review at a later time. Most vendors of epilepsy monitoring equipment have abandoned tape recordings.

Chapter 3.
Montages and
Localization

Montages were briefly introduced in the previous chapter. Here, we will discuss montages and localization in more detail. Modern EEG equipment allows for changing of montage on the fly, and for review of the same epoch in multiple montages for comparison. This is only part of the post-processing which can be performed on EEG recordings.

Referential montages

In referential recordings a single reference or two references (as in ipsilateral ear reference recordings) will be in the second input of each channel, while active electrodes are in the first input. In the ideal situation where the reference is neutral, potentials of interest are compared by amplitude, the largest amplitude reflecting the center of the field. However, references are frequently not neutral, hence the importance of considering more suitable references. With digital EEG recordings, this task is facilitated as the same potential can be examined with a variety of references. Thoughtful consideration of the most appropriate reference is necessary.

The average reference is derived from averaging the activity of all electrodes (except frontopolar and anterior temporal, which are subject to large eye movement artifacts). Assuming that no large field synchronous activity is present, there is cancellation based on cerebral activity being out of phase in different channels. The average reference is ideal for any focal abnormality. However, when discharges have a wide field, the average reference may become contaminated. Therefore, the average reference is not ideal for examining generalized spike-and-wave discharges and other generalized abnormalities.

The ipsilateral ear reference or linked ear reference is optimal for evaluation of generalized discharges, which tend to have the lowest amplitude in the temporal periphery. The ear reference is not suitable for temporal lobe discharges since the ear can be considered a lateral-basal temporal electrode. It is frequently involved in temporal lobe discharges. The average reference will usually be a more appropriate reference for studying temporal lobe activity. However, if the temporal lobe activity has a wide field, the average reference could also become contaminated. Using the midline (Cz, Fz or Pz) is useful, particularly for evaluating ictal activity if the ictal discharge has not involved the midline. In particular, if the discharge field is anterior, Pz could be sufficiently distant to be neutral. In contrast, if the ictal discharge is predominantly posterior, then Fz would be more appropriate. In some instances, the average reference can be manipulated to become neutral by excluding affected electrodes from the average.

Laplacian referential montage is excellent for identifying focal gradients by using a unique reference for each electrode, weighted by surrounding electrodes. The Laplacian montage is excellent for pointing out small focal potentials with a steep gradient, but is not appropriate for displaying generalized activity.

Localization in a referential montage

Localization in a referential montage is dependent on amplitude, assuming the presence of a neutral reference. The channel containing the highest amplitude will represent the location at the center of the field. Unfortunately, there is no ideal reference that is always neutral. For very focal discharges, the average reference is very suitable, because the contribution of the focal discharge to the average is greatly diluted by the uninvolved electrodes.

Bipolar Montages

Bipolar montages are composed of chains linking adjacent electrodes. These chains are either longitudinal, or transverse. They may also be in an arc, circle, or semicircle. The longitudinal bipolar montage (also called double banana) can be organized in several ways. The example listed is one of several acceptable arrangements. It is a general (but not universally followed) convention that anterior should be ahead of posterior and left ahead of right. Besides the example displayed in the table, one acceptable alternative arrangement is left temporal, left parasagittal, midline, right parasagittal, right temporal, and another arrangement is left temporal, right temporal, left parasagittal, right parasagittal, midline. There are relatively fewer permutations in the arrangement of transverse bipolar montage. Before digital EEG machines allowed expansion of the number of channels, the transverse bipolar montage did not include channels 1, 3, 18, and 20 below.

Localization of EEG activity in bipolar montages is by reversal of polarity (see below) and is optimally accomplished when the center of the field is within the chain. As a result, EEG activity centered in the frontal or occipital pole is not optimally assessed by either the longitudinal bipolar or transverse bipolar montage. This is where a circumferential montage may be useful. In a circumferential montage, the frontopolar and occipital electrodes are at the center of the anterior and posterior semicircular chains.

Localization of potentials in a bipolar montage

In a bipolar montage localization is accomplished by identification of reversal of polarity. Below are five situations and the expected pattern with each. EEG samples associated with each of these are presented immediately following this list.

- *Potential is present in a single electrode*: In this situation, there will be reversal of polarity between the two channels that have this electrode in common. (Example A)
- *Potential present equally at two electrodes*. Both involved electrodes are contained within the chain and not at the end of the chain: The channel that compares the two affected electrodes would show cancellation. The reversal of polarity will be seen across that channel. One can state that there is a reversal of polarity across a zone of equipotentiality between electrodes B and C. The two channels showing a deflection will be mirror images of each other, again with equal amplitude of opposite polarity. (Example B)

- *Potential at two electrodes, unequally involved.* Each involved electrode is contained within the chain, and not at the end of the chain. There will be reversal of polarity seen between the two channels that contain the most affected electrode. The potential will also be seen in the channel containing the less affected electrode and the unaffected electrode adjacent to it. The amplitude in the channel with the largest deflection will be equal to the sum of the amplitudes in the two channels with smaller deflections. From this, one can conclude that if there is a reversal of polarity that is not a mirror image, it indicates that there is involvement of more than a single electrode. (Example C)
- *Potential at the end of the chain.* Potential is present at the end of the chain and not involving any other electrode in the chain: In this instance there will be no reversal of polarity. A deflection will be seen in the first (or last) channel of the chain, where the potential is contained. (Examples D1 and D2)
- *Potential at the end of chain and adjacent electrode.* The potential involves one end of the chain and the electrode adjacent to it, equally: There will be cancellation in the channel that contains the two affected electrodes. The channel next to it will show a deflection. There will be no deflection in subsequent channels. There will be no reversal of polarity. (Example E)

As the last examples show, a potential that does not reverse polarity in a bipolar chain is not only involving the end of the chain, but involving the end of the chain maximally.

Montage localization examples

Example A: EEG potential at a single electrode.

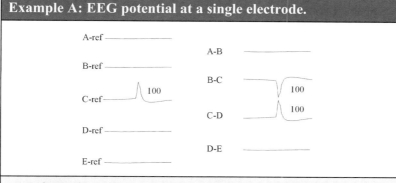

Referential recording to the left, corresponding bipolar recording to the right

Electrode C is the only affected electrode. The number next to the potential is a measure of amplitude. The bipolar recording shows reversal of polarity at C, the electrode in common between the second and third channels on the right. Note that B-C and C-D are mirror images, and the amplitude of the deflection is similar, but of opposite polarity.

Example B: EEG potential at two electrodes, equally involved.

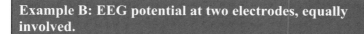
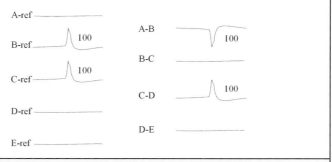

Since electrodes B and C are equally affected, the difference between them is 0, hence the flat line. There is a reversal of polarity across a zone of equipotentiality between B and C. B and C are equipotential, i.e. equally affected.

Example C: EEG potential at two electrodes, unequally involved.

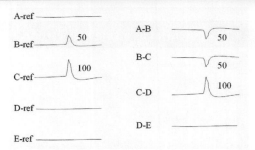

This illustrates how EEG is a an arithmetic operation. The reversal of polarity at C indicates that the highest voltage is at C. The finding of a lower amplitude at B-C than C-D suggests that there is involvement of B.

Example D1: EEG potential at the end of chain.

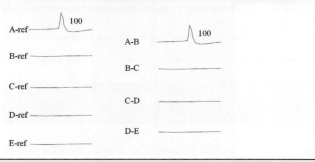

End of chain phenomenon. The potential originates in the anterior end of the chain.

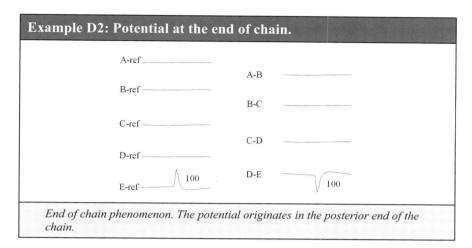

Example D2: Potential at the end of chain.

End of chain phenomenon. The potential originates in the posterior end of the chain.

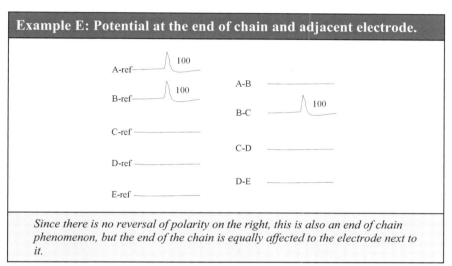

Example E: Potential at the end of chain and adjacent electrode.

Since there is no reversal of polarity on the right, this is also an end of chain phenomenon, but the end of the chain is equally affected to the electrode next to it.

Every pattern in a bipolar montage has several potential solutions in a referential montage, assuming a neutral reference. Usually, one solution is the most likely. (See examples on page 36.)

Consider the following two figures together. The bipolar recording on the left side of each figure is identical. On the right is a potential referential recording, which could correspond to the bipolar recording.

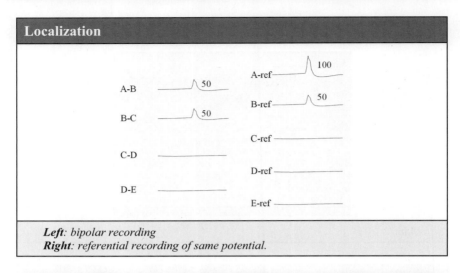

Left: *bipolar recording*
Right: *referential recording of same potential.*

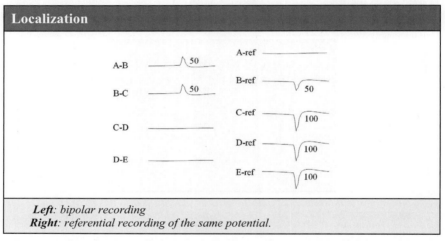

Left: *bipolar recording*
Right: *referential recording of the same potential.*

Which of these two possibilities is most likely? In these examples, the bottom possibility is less likely, because it assumes that three electrodes are all equally affected. Therefore, the top possibility is more likely.

Although a bipolar montage can be used to suggest asymmetries in widespread activity, these asymmetries have to be confirmed in a referential montage. The main reason for that is that each bipolar channel is an arithmetic subtraction of adjacent active electrodes. There will be a low amplitude if adjacent electrodes are almost equally affected. The presence of a high amplitude depends on a sharp gradient between adjacent electrodes. Fortunately, most potentials have the highest gradients near the center of the field, but this is not always the case. The examples below illustrate this point. In addition, an electrical bridge due to electrode paste smear will produce a very low amplitude that could be misinterpreted as attenuation of activity in that region.

Localization with referential recording

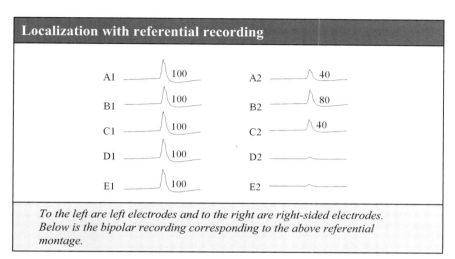

To the left are left electrodes and to the right are right-sided electrodes. Below is the bipolar recording corresponding to the above referential montage.

Localization with bipolar recording

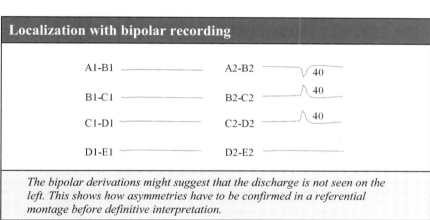

The bipolar derivations might suggest that the discharge is not seen on the left. This shows how asymmetries have to be confirmed in a referential montage before definitive interpretation.

Localization with referential and bipolar montages.

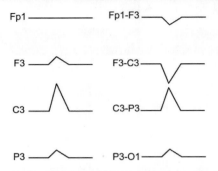

Left: *A referential montage is used where the reference is over an inactive area. The sharp wave has a maximum at C3 but the field can be seen at F3 and P3. FP1 and O1 (not shown) are not in the field of the sharp wave.*

Right: *Bipolar montage, the left parasagittal portion of the longitudinal bipolar montage.*

For optimal localization, a discharge may need to be studied in more than one montage. The DVD provides many examples of how the appearance of potentials is changed by the montage. It will provide some guidance as to how to select the optimal montage for evaluation of electrical transients and seizures.

Chapter 4.
EEG Analysis

Terminology

The following terms are essential for describing EEG activity:

Rhythmic: term used to describe ongoing EEG activity composed of recurring waves of equal duration. The waves need not be identical, but they usually resemble each other. Cerebral activity is never perfect, and slight variation should be allowed. For example, the activity below is rhythmic, but some individual waves are slightly shorter or longer than others, as demonstrated in the second example.

Rhythm

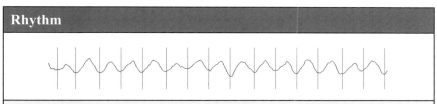

The vertical lines mark individual waves. Although there is a minor variation in wave duration and appearance, waves are fairly similar.

Rhythm: EEG activity composed of recurring waves of equal duration. A rhythm is often characterized by its frequency.

Frequency: This indicates the number of individual waves that could fit into one second. Frequency is measured in Hertz (Hz) or cycles per second (cps). The two mean the same thing, but Hz is preferable. Frequency can be applied to single waves as well as to a rhythm. If applied to a single wave, it is calculated based on the following formula: frequency (Hz) = 1/wavelength (seconds). Most digital EEG manufacturers will provide automatic calculation of frequency by marking the margins of a wave. For a rhythm, the frequency will express how many waves actually fit in one second. In the example on page 40, nine waves can be counted between the two one-second lines . The frequency can also be derived with the formula above. The duration of the average wave is 111 msec or 0.111 sec. The frequency is 1/0.111= 9 Hz. Frequency determination of fast activity can be made more reliably by counting waves contained in one second, because of slight variation in wavelength duration.

Regular rhythm

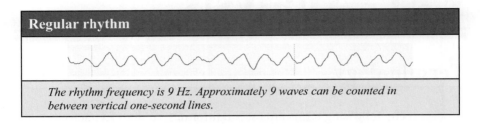

The rhythm frequency is 9 Hz. Approximately 9 waves can be counted in between vertical one-second lines.

Regular: Applies to activity that is uniform, with individual waves having fairly consistent shape, in addition to fairly consistent duration. Thus activity that is regular will also be rhythmic. Most rhythmic activity will also be regular, although this is not always the case. Regular activity is sometimes referred to as *monomorphic*.

Irregular: Activity that is not uniform. It is in theory possible for rhythmic activity to be irregular, but that is uncommon.

Arrhythmic: Term used to describe ongoing EEG activity composed of waves of unequal duration. Below are two examples of arrhythmic activity. In this activity individual wave components have differing wavelengths. Arrhythmic activity is also irregular. Note that individual waves not only have unequal duration, but also unequal shape and unequal amplitude. This is often called *polymorphic*.

Arrhythmic activity

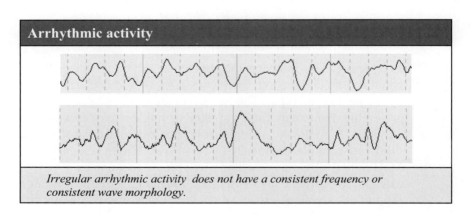

Irregular arrhythmic activity does not have a consistent frequency or consistent wave morphology.

Activity such as shown in the figure on page 40 can be continuous or intermittent. If the activity is intermittent, it can be described as rare, occasional, moderately frequent, very frequent, or almost continuous. However, it is most useful to indicate the percentage of time that the activity is present.

Transient: a wave or combination of waves that stands out from the surrounding background. A transient can be normal or abnormal.

Complex: combination of 2 or more waves. This combination will usually be consistent when the complex recurs. Below is a polyspike-and-wave complex that includes a series of 3 spikes followed by a high voltage slow wave.

Complex

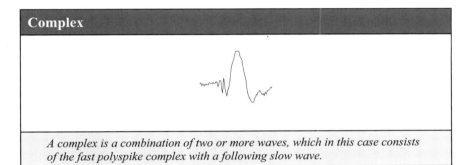

A complex is a combination of two or more waves, which in this case consists of the fast polyspike complex with a following slow wave.

Analysis of the complex

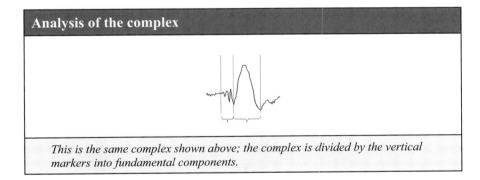

This is the same complex shown above; the complex is divided by the vertical markers into fundamental components.

The examples that follow show a series of spike-and-wave complexes demonstrating that complexes look fairly consistent when they recur.

Spike-and-wave complex

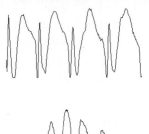

Although the two examples above vary in appearance from each other, recurrent complexes in each example are fairly consistent. Both have a classic appearance of spike and wave complexes, with well-formed spikes and associated slow waves.

Periodic: term used to describe transients or complexes that recur, but with intervening activity in between them. The incidence or rate of recurrence of periodic transients is less than the *frequency* of this transient determined as 1/wavelength. The illustration on page 43 demonstrates the difference between rhythmic and periodic discharges. The bottom line shows a single transient. The top line shows the same transient recurring as a periodic discharge. The middle line shows the same transient recurring as a rhythmic train.

Periodic pattern.

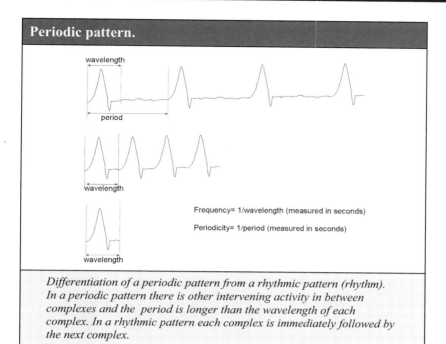

Frequency= 1/wavelength (measured in seconds)

Periodicity= 1/period (measured in seconds)

Differentiation of a periodic pattern from a rhythmic pattern (rhythm). In a periodic pattern there is other intervening activity in between complexes and the period is longer than the wavelength of each complex. In a rhythmic pattern each complex is immediately followed by the next complex.

Spatial distribution. The electrodes involved with a discharge and the degree of their involvement determines the field. Discharges can be described as focal, regional, lateralized, or generalized. Focal discharges are restricted to a few electrodes on one side. The term regional can be applied to a discharge that is involving more than a few electrodes. If electrodes on one side are all affected, the discharge can be considered lateralized. Generalized discharges affect all electrodes, on both sides. It is almost never the case that all electrodes are affected equally. Many generalized discharges have voltage predominance anteriorly, but there can be voltage predominance in a variety of regions. The terms *diffuse* and *widespread* are sometimes used synonymously with *generalized*, but generally indicate a less clearly generalized field. For focal and regional discharges a field can be designated with isopotential lines that join equally affected regions.

On page 44 is an example of a field. The center of the field is at F3, then C3 is a bit less involved, followed by Fp1 and F7, then Fz, Cz, and P3.

Spatial distribution of a potential

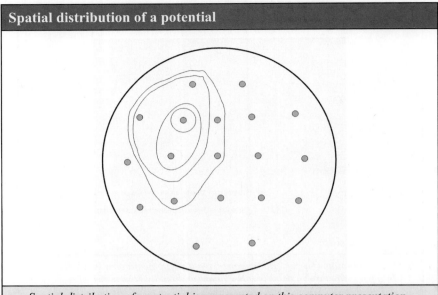

Spatial distribution of a potential is represented on this computer presentation. This is a standard view of the scalp and the lines represent potential isobars.

Timing: When discharges are seen in several locations, then the temporal relationship of the activity in these different regions can be described with the following terms: *sychronous* and *asynchronous.*

Synchronous: occurring in two regions simultaneously. To indicate that a discharge is occurring on the two sides simultaneously, the terms "bisynchronous" or "bilaterally synchronous" are frequently used.

The example on page 45 shows a bilaterally synchronous spike-and-wave discharge. It is easiest to see how the spikes are simultaneous on the two sides.

Synchronous spike-and-wave discharge

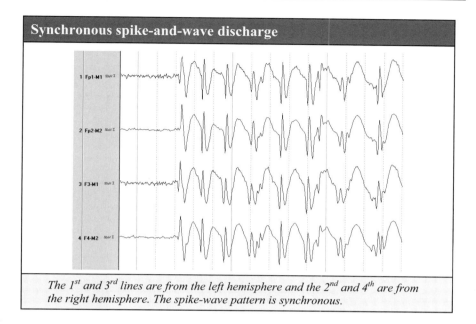

The 1ˢᵗ and 3ʳᵈ lines are from the left hemisphere and the 2ⁿᵈ and 4ᵗʰ are from the right hemisphere. The spike-wave pattern is synchronous.

Asynchronous: describes transients or other activity that is seen in several regions, but not simultaneously. "Independent" is often applied to a more extreme situation where discharges occur at different times in two or more regions, or on the two sides.

The circled discharges on page 46 are occurring independently on the two sides and in different regions on the same side.

Asynchronous discharges

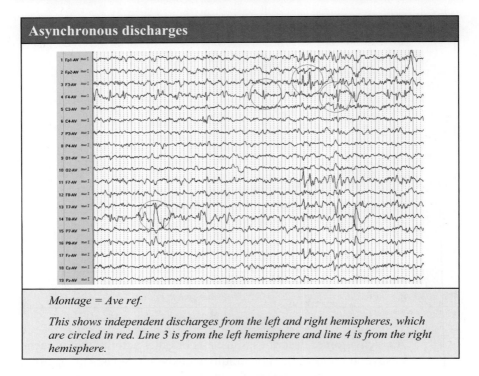

Montage = Ave ref.

This shows independent discharges from the left and right hemispheres, which are circled in red. Line 3 is from the left hemisphere and line 4 is from the right hemisphere.

The tracing below shows both independent and bisynchronous discharges.

Independent and bisynchronous discharges

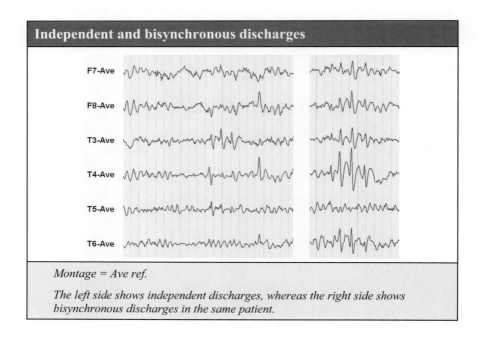

Montage = Ave ref.

The left side shows independent discharges, whereas the right side shows bisynchronous discharges in the same patient.

Synchronous activity can be in phase, indicating a perfect correspondence in time, or out of phase, indicating a small delay on one side in comparison with the other. When there is a horizontal dipole, with negativity in one region and positivity in another, the discharge is out of phase in these two regions.

Basic EEG analysis

EEG rhythms are divided into four frequency bands for descriptive purposes. Each rhythm is not specifically normal or abnormal, but the interpretation depends on the context. For example, alpha activity in the occipital region is normal in an awake patient with eyes closed. The same frequency activity is very abnormal when diffusely distributed in a comatose patient.

EEG rhythms

Rhythm	Frequency	Normal examples	Abnormal examples
Alpha	8-13 Hz	Waking posterior rhythm in older children and adults. Mu rhythm	Alpha coma. Seizure activity in the alpha range
Beta	> 13 Hz	Drowsiness in children.	Drug-induced. Breach rhythm over a skull defect. Seizure onset in the beta range.
Theta	4-7 Hz	Drowsiness, young children; temporal theta in the elderly	Structural lesion. Encephalopathy.
Delta	< 4 Hz	Sleep, posterior slow waves of youth.	Focal structural lesion. Encephalopathy.

Fundamental frequency bands

Alpha

Alpha rhythm is 8-13 Hz. It is most commonly seen in normal patients from the occipital regions in the awake state with eyes closed. When the eyes open, the alpha rhythm is attenuated. Because the occipital rhythm is in the alpha range, the term *alpha rhythm* is used for the *posterior dominant rhythm.* Therefore, one need keep in mind the dual meaning of this term. There are other EEG activities in the alpha range: the "Mu rhythm," which is the resting rhythm of the rolandic region, and the "third rhythm," which is seen at times in the temporal region.

Beta

Beta rhythm is greater than 13 Hz, and is most often seen in patients who have been sedated with benzodiazepines and barbiturates. The beta component of the rhythm should be commented on during interpretation of the record, and an association with concurrent medications should be considered. However, beta can be abnormal, so the rhythm cannot be overlooked.

Theta

Theta rhythm is 4-7.9 Hz and is seen most commonly in normal drowsiness and in children. Theta in normal children makes determination of subtle encephalopathy difficult. Theta is most likely to be abnormal if it is the posterior dominant rhythm in a waking adult, or if it is focal.

Delta

Delta activity is less than 4 Hz and is most commonly seen in sleep. There is a gradual increase in the amount of delta activity as the patient progresses from stage 2 to stage 3 and stage 4 sleep. Focal delta activity develops in patients with focal structural lesions, and a variable and unusual appearance creates the name *polymorphic delta activity*. Rhythmic anterior or posterior delta activity can be seen in patients with diffuse or metabolic disorders, as *frontal intermittent rhythmic delta activity* (FIRDA) or *occipital intermittent rhythmic delta activity* (OIRDA).

Transients

Spikes and sharp waves

Spikes and sharp waves are the terms used when sharp transients are determined to be abnormal and suggestive of epilepsy. Spikes and sharp waves are also referred to as interictal epileptiform discharges/activity. Spikes have a duration of less than 70 msec and sharp waves have a duration of 70-200 msec, therefore appearing less sharp than spikes. Combinations of spikes, sharp waves, and slow waves are also epileptiform discharges.

Spikes and sharp waves generated at the crown of a gyrus are usually surface negative, with the positive end of the dipole deep to the cortex. However, some spike foci have a horizontal dipole, where both the positive and negative poles are seen on surface recordings. One notable example is Rolandic epilepsy where the positive end of the dipole can be seen anteriorly.

There are a number of features that distinguish spikes and sharp waves from nonepileptiform sharp transients. Epileptiform discharges are different from the surrounding activity. They tend to be of high voltage, they are usually asymmetrical with a longer and larger second half in comparison with the first half, they tend to have more than one phase, and they tend to have an after-going slow wave (see figure). In addition, epileptiform discharges are more convincing if they arise from an abnormal background. Epileptiform discharges should be different from normal sharp activity (such as vertex waves) in field and in the state of arousal of the patient.

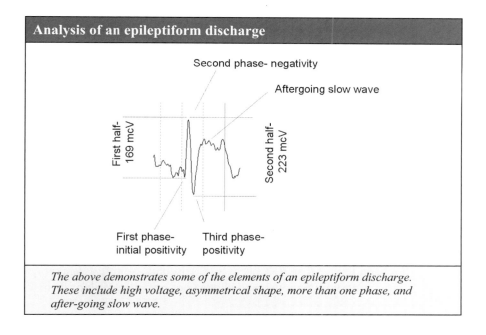

Analysis of an epileptiform discharge

Second phase- negativity

Aftergoing slow wave

First half- 169 mcV

Second half- 223 mcV

First phase- initial positivity

Third phase- positivity

The above demonstrates some of the elements of an epileptiform discharge. These include high voltage, asymmetrical shape, more than one phase, and after-going slow wave.

Spike-like potentials that are normal are frequently a source of over-interpretation. Sharp potentials that are often over-interpreted include sharp physiologic activity such as is seen with skull defects, EMG potentials, and artifact. Differentiation of spikes and sharp waves from nonepileptiform potentials may also take into consideration the consistency of appearance of epileptiform discharges.

Non-epileptiform sharp activity

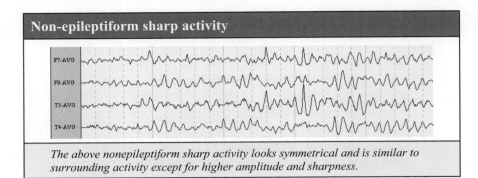

The above nonepileptiform sharp activity looks symmetrical and is similar to surrounding activity except for higher amplitude and sharpness.

Lateral rectus spikes

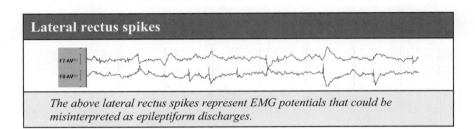

The above lateral rectus spikes represent EMG potentials that could be misinterpreted as epileptiform discharges.

Epileptiform discharges do not consistently have a strong association with epilepsy. Caution should be used in the interpretation of pediatric EEGs with occipital or rolandic sharp waves. Caution should also be exercised in the final interpretation if only a single spike is recorded during the whole EEG.

Sharply contoured slow waves

These are transients that could have been sharp waves had they not been longer that 200 msec. Such discharges have a weaker association with epilepsy and should not be called epileptiform.

Slow waves

Slow wave transients can be in the theta or delta range, and stand out from the background. Focal slow transients can be a sign of focal CNS damage or reversible dysfunction (see Chapter 1). Focal slow activity can occasionally be the only abnormality seen in association with focal epilepsy.

Epileptiform transients		
Transient	Duration	Variants
Spike	25-70 ms	Spike-and-wave complex; polyspike complex; polyspike-and-wave complex
Sharp wave	70-200 ms	Sharp-and-slow-wave complex; multiple-sharp-and-slow-wave complex
Sharply contoured slow wave (strictly not epileptiform)	>200 ms	

Spike

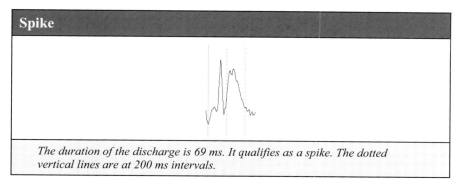

The duration of the discharge is 69 ms. It qualifies as a spike. The dotted vertical lines are at 200 ms intervals.

Sharp wave

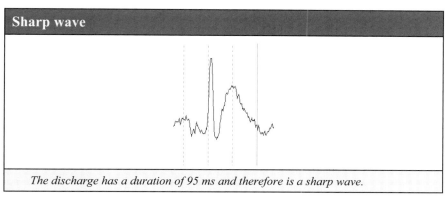

The discharge has a duration of 95 ms and therefore is a sharp wave.

Sharp wave

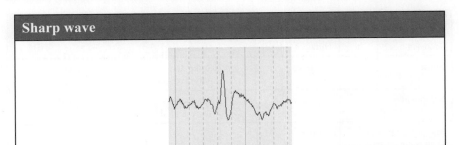

This discharge is also a sharp wave. Even though it has an after-going slow wave, it is not called a sharp-and-slow-wave complex unless the slow wave has a high amplitude – usually at least as high as the sharp wave.

Spike-and-wave complex

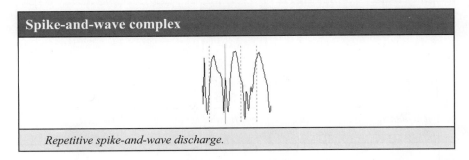

Repetitive spike-and-wave discharge.

Polyspike-and-wave complex

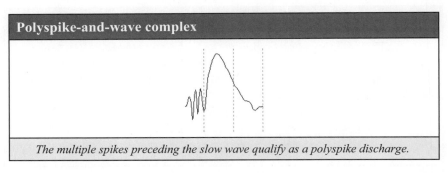

The multiple spikes preceding the slow wave qualify as a polyspike discharge.

Clinical analysis and interpretation

Review of routine EEG

Some neurophysiologists begin with review of the EEG before any of the clinical information is reviewed. However, most of us prefer to know the clinical details including the age of the patient, reason for the study, current medications, and technician's impression of the state.

Review includes determination of the following:

- Background rhythm
- Topographical organization of the background activities
- Transients
- State changes
- Response to activation methods

Particular attention is paid to the following:

- Ictal activity
- Sharp waves or spikes
- Focal and generalized slow activity
- Inappropriate response to stimuli
- EEG correlates to changes in state or behavior

It is usually best to proceed with one uninterrupted rapid review of the recording before returning to it for a more detailed and in-depth assessment. The reason for this is that there may be a prominent abnormality later in the recording that would make subtle or uncertain findings less important to make a decision on.

Review of video EEG

Video EEG is initially reviewed by the technician. It is unrealistic for the neurophysiologist to review every epoch of the video EEG. The key epochs reviewed include the ones thought to be of interest by the technician and ones that were noted by the event marker. In our institution, a spike and seizure detection program is operated on line and identifies suspected seizures as well as spikes and sharp waves. In addition, the patient and patient's family are instructed to push an event marker button, which leaves a mark on the EEG recording. The technologist reviews all the patient events and computer seizure detections, and marks all the seizures, as well as suspected ictal discharges. The electroencephalographer reviews these segments first, analyzing both the EEG discharges and the clinical seizure semiology. In addition, the electroencephalographer will usually review the spike detections and time samples (usually about 5 minutes per hour).

Guidelines to clinical interpretation

Clinical interpretation of EEG should take into account not only the EEG recording but also the clinical information that was provided. Unfortunately, this information can be quite limited, which limits the utility of the interpretation. As with all neurophysiologic interpretations, the EEG report represents a type of consultation. Therefore, the impression should not only be descriptive but also clinically useful.

An EEG report impression could read:

> Abnormal study because of generalized asynchronous irregular theta and delta activity.

Such an interpretation may not be useful to the referring clinician.

The impression should include a summary of the key findings as well as a clinical interpretation. These could be divided into two paragraphs, as below

> *EEG Diagnosis*: Abnormal study because of generalized asynchronous irregular theta and delta activity. No focal findings were seen.

> *Clinical Interpretation*: This EEG consistent with a generalized encephalopathy, but is not specific as to etiology.

The impression is not a substitute for a description of the record. The body of the report would include a description of the record including background, state changes, and presence and absence of normal and abnormal rhythms or transients. Any epileptiform and focal abnormalities, abnormal responses or absence of response should be described. The clinical interpretation may need to be tailored to the question asked. For example, if the clinical question is "rule out status epilepticus," it would be helpful for the clinical interpretation to add "there was no seizure activity."

Epilepsy monitoring unit reports follow the same guidelines. In our center, the report includes, in addition to identifying information, the following:

- A preamble summarizing the background information and the reason for the study
- A description of the baseline EEG (this is like a standard EEG with hyperventilation and photic stimulation, performed within the first day of admission),
- A daily description of clinical seizures and their electrographic correlate
- A daily description of the interictal abnormalities
- EEG diagnosis summarizing the key abnormalities, starting with ictal discharges (focusing on localization at onset), then interictal discharges, then nonepileptiform abnormalities

- Clinical interpretation. In this section, the clinical seizure description is provided first, with a statement about the localizing and lateralizing value of the seizure signs, then a statement about how the semiology agrees with the EEG ictal onset and other EEG abnormalities, and then a summary synthesis of all the findings, to provide a seizure diagnosis, classification, lateralization, and localization, together with the degree of certainty of these determinations.

Chapter 5.
Normal Routine EEG

Adult

Routine EEG usually begins with the patient awake with the eyes closed. The technician asks the patient to open and close the eyes to assess the posterior background rhythm and its reactivity. If activation methods are used, they are performed during the initial segment of the EEG. Finally, the patient is allowed to rest, progress into drowsiness and possibly fall asleep. Evaluation of encephalopathy does not typically require a sleeping study, but evaluation for seizures is best if a sleep study is performed.

Waking

Adults with the eyes closed have a posterior dominant rhythm of about 10 Hz. The minimum allowable frequency is 8.5 Hz, and 11 Hz is the upper end of the range. Anterior cerebral EEG shows low-voltage fast activity. Eye movement artifact is superimposed. A frontal-predominant beta activity is seen when patients are sedated with benzodiazepines or barbiturates, but this is less prominent with chloral hydrate.

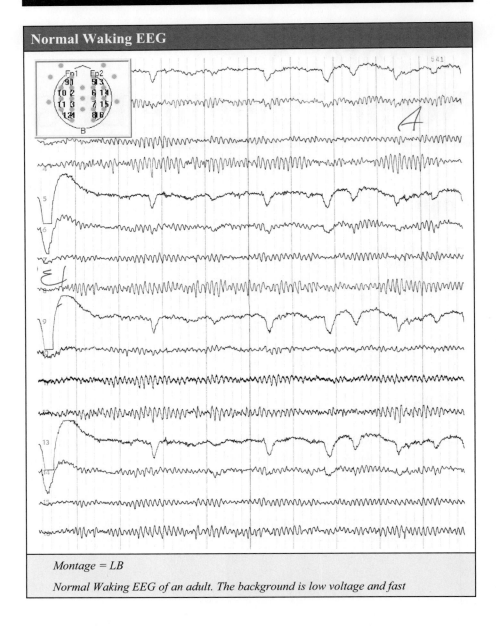

Normal Waking EEG

Montage = LB

Normal Waking EEG of an adult. The background is low voltage and fast

Digital EEG analysis shows a small amount of theta and delta during the awake state, but this is not prominent with visual analysis. Older patients have less prominent posterior dominant alpha activity. Also, tense patients may have little or no visible posterior dominant alpha-range activity. This should be commented on in the report, but not interpreted as an abnormality in the absence of other findings.

Eye closure results in attenuation of the posterior dominant rhythm, as shown in the figure.

Effect of eye opening on posterior dominant rhythm.

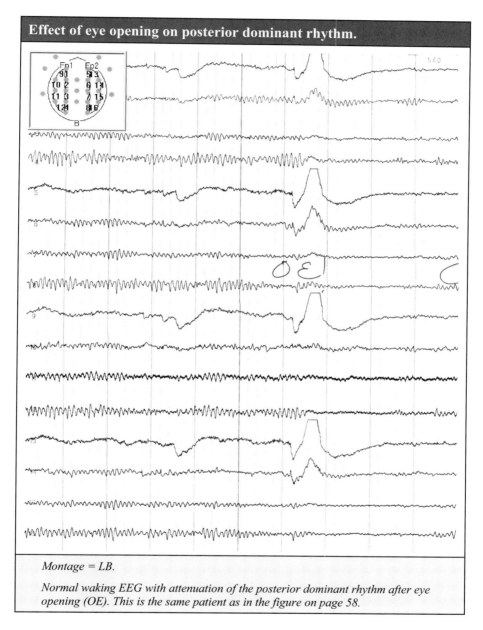

Montage = LB.

Normal waking EEG with attenuation of the posterior dominant rhythm after eye opening (OE). This is the same patient as in the figure on page 58.

Drowsiness

Patients progress from waking to drowsiness, during which time there are several changes, including progressive reduction of muscle artifact, a slight reduction in the posterior rhythm frequency (usually not more than 1 Hz), anterior widening of the field of posterior dominant rhythm, and slow horizontal eye movements (SEM). This is sleep stage 1A. With progression to stage 1B, there is attenuation then loss of posterior dominant rhythm. The posterior dominant rhythm is reduced to less than 20% with the appearance of theta.

Vertex waves may be seen in stage 1B, but this is more of a characteristic of stage 2 sleep. Theta becomes more prominent. Differentiation of stages 1A from 1B is not important for routine EEG, but is important in sleep studies, as 3 consecutive epochs (1 epoch=30 seconds) of stage IB is considered the onset of sleep.

Sleeping

Stage 2: Sleep is most easily recognized in stage 2. Stage 2 sleep is heralded by the presence of sleep spindles, more prominent vertex waves, and K-complexes, which are longer polyphasic vertex waves often associated with spindle activity. There is complete loss of the posterior dominant alpha rhythm. Since vertex waves may appear in drowsiness and sleep stage 1B, the main differentiating feature of stage 2 is the appearance of sleep spindles. Delta begins to appear at this stage.

Stage 2 sleep

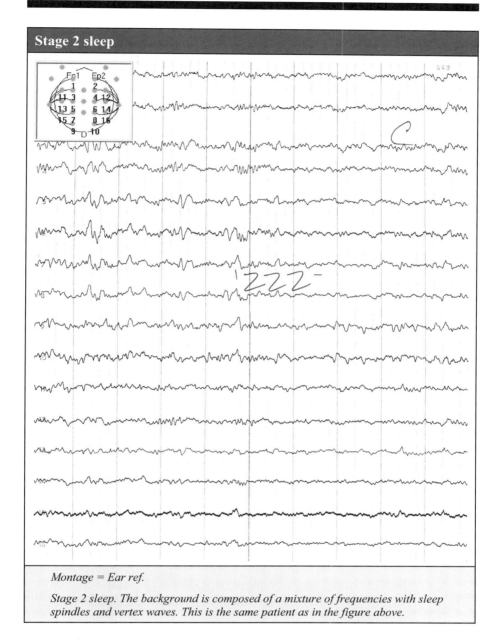

Montage = Ear ref.

Stage 2 sleep. The background is composed of a mixture of frequencies with sleep spindles and vertex waves. This is the same patient as in the figure above.

Stage 3: Stage 3 sleep is characterized by more delta and fewer faster frequencies. Delta comprises 20-50% of the record. Stage 3 sleep is not commonly seen in routine office EEG.

Stage 4: Delta activity predominates in stage 4 sleep, which now comprises more than 50% of the record. Vertex waves and sleep spindles are often absent. Stage 4 sleep is rarely seen on routine office EEG.

Wake and sleep stages	
Stage	Features
Waking	PDR of 8.5-11 Hz, desynchronized background.
Stage 1A	Reduction of muscle artifact, anterior widening of the field of posterior dominant rhythm, slow horizontal eye movements (SEM).
Stage 1B	Attenuation of the PDR. Appearance of theta activity. Vertex waves may appear
Stage 2	Loss of the PDR. Sleep spindles. Vertex waves and K-complexes.
Stage 3	More delta activity (20-50% of EEG). Fewer vertex waves and spindles. Spindles become more anterior and slower in frequency.
Stage 4	Prominent delta (>50% of EEG). Vertex waves and spindles are few to none.
REM sleep	Low-voltage fast background with rapid eye movements.

REM: Rapid eye movement sleep is characterized by a low-voltage fast background. Superficially, this pattern may resemble drowsiness, but is differentiated by rapid eye movements, hypotonia on submental EMG, and irregular respiratory rate.

Progression of sleep stages: Waking, drowsiness, and stage 2 sleep are commonly seen in routine office EEG. The progression is from waking to stage 1A to stage 1B to stage 2. With prolonged recordings, patients may progress to stage 3 then 4. The progression to stage 4 does not occur with each cycle. There are three to five cycles in a night's sleep. REM sleep occurs after at least one sleep cycle, and is of increased duration with later cycles.

Children

The EEG in children is superficially similar to that in adults in that there is a posterior dominant rhythm that is attenuated and eventually replaced by slower activity in drowsiness and sleep. There are important differences, which are age and state dependent.

Waking

Posterior rhythm: The normal waking background of the child depends on age. The posterior dominant rhythm is approximately 4 Hz in the infant and becomes faster throughout childhood, reaching 8 Hz by age 3, and the average adult frequency of 10 Hz by 10 years of age. The figure below shows the maturation of the posterior dominant rhythm. The amplitude tends to be higher than in adults, in the range of 50-100 µV.

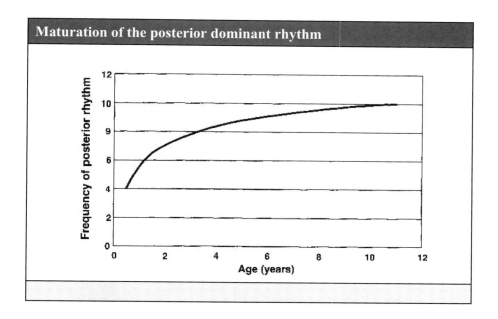

Maturation of the posterior dominant rhythm

Activation maneuvers: In addition to differences in frequency composition of the native waking background, there are also differences in response to activation maneuvers. Hyperventilation produces higher amplitude slow activity in children than in adults. Photic stimulation can produce alerting at any age, but it is not uncommon for children to go to sleep during photic stimulation.

Posterior slow waves of youth: There are slow waves superimposed on and intermixed with the normal posterior waking background, referred to as slow waves of youth. These could potentially be confused with abnormal slow potentials indicating encephalopathy, especially in the young child with a posterior rhythm in the theta range. Posterior slow waves may have an episodic occurrence or may be seen sequentially. They are usually notched, suggesting that several alpha waves have merged to form them. They are not usually confused with epileptiform activity, although the sequence of an alpha wave followed by a slow wave occasionally suggests a sharp and slow wave complex.

In addition to posterior slow waves, there is more theta anteriorly in young children than in adults, and this, also, should not be interpreted as abnormal.

Neurophysiologists who are not accustomed to interpretation of children's EEGs often misinterpret normal slow activity as pathological slow activity, indicative of encephalopathy. Therefore, consideration must be made to age as well as the state of the patient.

Drowsiness

One pattern of drowsiness seen in early childhood is that of generalized bisynchronous high voltage slow waves, often appearing abruptly. This pattern referred to a hypnagogic hypersynchrony. It becomes less frequent with advancing age, and is no longer seen by adolescence.

Sleeping

Sleep should be obtained when the clinical question is seizures, since interictal discharges (and sometimes ictal discharges) are more common in sleep. For some patients, abnormal electrical activity is only seen in sleep.

There is effectively no difference between sedated sleep and natural sleep, so there should be no hesitation to administer sedatives to patients in the EEG lab during the day. Chloral hydrate is most commonly used since there is a wide safety margin and this agent does not produce the prominent drug-induced beta activity which is typical of benzodiazepines and barbiturates. However, this is considered conscious sedation and requires monitoring of vital signs.

The sleep records of children and adults are more alike than the waking records. However, there are maturational changes in children. In addition sleep activity of children can be particularly sharp and high in voltage.

Vertex waves: Vertex waves are not present at birth, but begin to appear at about 5 months of age. By 2 years of age they are prominent in stage 2 sleep, sharp in configuration, and high amplitude. They can be so prominent as to be confused with epileptiform activity.

Sleep spindles: Sleep spindles are also not present at birth, but begin to appear consistently at about 2 months. The early sleep spindles are often prolonged and have an appearance different from adult spindles, in that that they have a sharp negative peak and rounded base. They are also frequently asynchronous or asymmetrical. After 18 months of age the majority of spindles should be synchronous. By 2 years of age, the general appearance of the sleep spindles is the same as in adults.

Cone waves. These high voltage occipital cone-shaped waves may be seen in the occipital regions in infancy.

Activation methods

Photic stimulation

Photic stimulation is produced by a bright strobe, which is placed in front of the patient with the eyes closed. The flashes are bright enough to illuminate the retina well through the eye lid.

Methods

The stimulation protocols are programmed into most modern EEG machines, but one typical protocol is the following:

- Train duration of 10 seconds
- Interval between trains of 10 seconds
- Initial flash rate of 3/sec
- Higher flash rates subsequently delivered up to 30/sec

Abnormal EEG activity elicited by a specific frequency should be identified by the technologist, and subsequently that particular frequency should be repeated at the end of the photic stimulation session, to verify that the response was not coincidental.

For safety reasons, it is not advisable to precipitate a full-fledged generalized tonic-clonic seizure with photic stimulation. If a clear photoconvulsive response appears, the technologist should abort the stimulation train before a seizure develops. If a consistent photoconvulsive response is noted at two to three consecutive frequencies, then stimulation can be resumed from the highest frequency to establish the upper limit of the photosensitivity frequency range.

Types of response

Responses to photic stimulation can be normal, abnormal, or artifactual. These are:

Normal:

- Visual evoked response
- Driving response

Abnormal:

- Photoconvulsive response

Artifact:

- Photoelectric artifact
- Photomyoclonic response

Visual evoked response (VER)

The visual evoked response is the same potential that is recorded during evoked potentials. The difference in appearance is because of the method of data display and the absence of averaging. The VER is seen with low flash frequencies, usually most prominent at and below 5/sec.

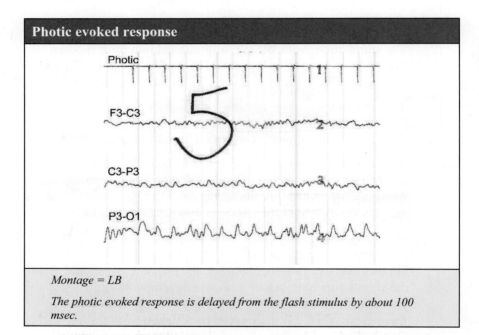

Photic evoked response

Photic

F3-C3

C3-P3

P3-O1

Montage = LB

The photic evoked response is delayed from the flash stimulus by about 100 msec.

The absence of a VER is not abnormal unless unilateral. Such asymmetry suggests abnormality in projections from one lateral geniculate to the cortex, of the calcarine cortex, itself.

Driving response

The driving response appears as the flash frequency accelerates beyond 7/sec, and the next evoked potential starts before the last evoked potential has ended. It is created by the visual evoked responses merging into each other. The driving response is usually most prominent at the frequency of the posterior rhythm, or at multiples thereof.

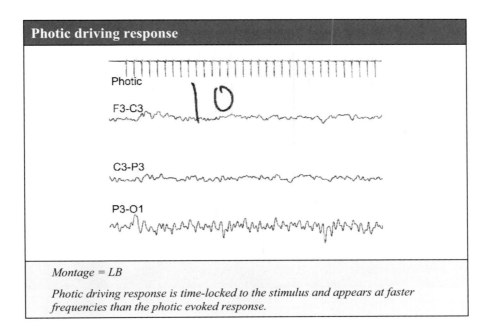

Photic driving response

Montage = LB

Photic driving response is time-locked to the stimulus and appears at faster frequencies than the photic evoked response.

The driving response is usually seen, but absence is not interpreted as an abnormality unless unilateral or markedly asymmetric in the absence of other abnormalities.

Photomyoclonic response

The photomyoclonic response is not cerebral in origin, but rather is electrical activity in the frontal scalp muscles, which is induced by the flash stimulus in susceptible individuals. Repeated contraction of these muscles produces EMG activity, which is time-locked to the stimulus, and recorded from the frontal leads. There is a delay of 50-60 msec between the flash and the EMG activity.

The main problem with the photomyoclonic response is in differentiation of this from photoconvulsive response. Some general guidelines are discussed in the following table.

Differentiation of photomyoclonic from photoconvulsive responses		
Feature	Photomyoclonic	Photoconvulsive
Spatial distribution	Anterior	Posterior or generalized
Termination	End of the stimulus	May stop before the end of the stimulus or outlast the end of the stimulus
Rise-time of the spike	Fast (EMG) spikes	Slower, spike-and-wave complexes most common
Frequency	Same frequency as the flash	Frequency is independent of the flash frequency, usually slower

Photoconvulsive response

The photoconvulsive response is a marker for seizure tendency, and most often noted with generalized epilepsies. Less commonly, photosensitivity is noted with partial epilepsy (occipital lobe epilepsy, and even less commonly temporal lobe epilepsy). While some patients will have already noticed that there is photic trigger of their seizures, this is not always the case. Some patients with photosensitivity have never had a spontaneous seizure.

Photoconvulsive response

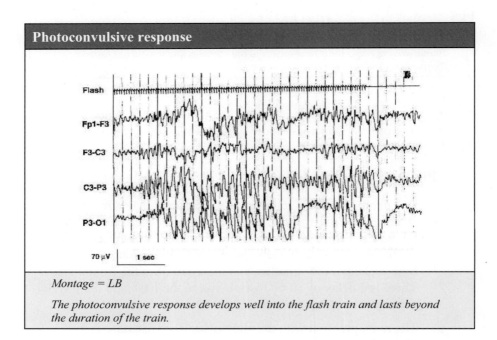

Montage = LB

The photoconvulsive response develops well into the flash train and lasts beyond the duration of the train.

The discharge is usually activated by a band of flash frequencies rather than by the entirety of the flash procedure. Identification of photoconvulsive response is generally by the following criteria:

- Activated by a band of flash rates
- Does not begin with the first flash in the train
- Frequency is not time-locked to the stimulus
- May outlast the photic stimulation train or stop before the end of the train

The photoconvulsive response is always interpreted as abnormal. It has been suggested that the best correlation with epilepsy occurs if the discharge outlasts the stimulus train; however, this has not been consistently noted.

Photoelectric artifact

The photoelectric artifact is non-cerebral and not EMG. The potential is generated by the electrode-gel complex. Light produces changes in the electrode that disturb subtle junction potentials between the electrode and gel. This release is detected mostly in the frontal electrodes that are directly illuminated as a rhythmic spike potential with a frequency equal to the frequency of photic stimulation.

The artifact is often contaminating insecure leads with high impedance, so there is not equal representation across the forehead, and loss of common mode rejection. It may be difficult to distinguish from the electroretinogram (ERG) activity that records potentials from the retina. The ERG is often seen in the frontopolar electrodes as well, at high gains, when there is a paucity of electrocerebral activity.

Hyperventilation

Hyperventilation is used predominantly to activate the 3-per-second spike-and-wave discharge of absence seizures. Patients with untreated childhood absence epilepsy will almost always have these discharges with hyperventilation. In some patients, the discharges are only seen during hyperventilation.

Hyperventilation

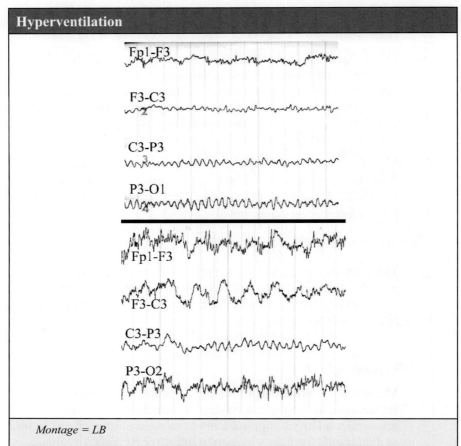

Fp1-F3

F3-C3

C3-P3

P3-O1

Fp1-F3

F3-C3

C3-P3

P3-O2

Montage = LB

Top: *Normal EEG in the awake state with a normal posterior dominant rhythm*

Bottom: *Hyperventilation results in increased muscle and movement artifact, and prominent slow activity, which is a normal finding.*

The normal response to hyperventilation is generalized slow activity, both synchronous and asynchronous. In adults, there is mostly appearance of theta range activity. The slow activity is more prominent in children than in adults and also more prominent and persistent in patients with hypoglycemia.

Hyperventilation is performed for 3 minutes on routine testing, and should be performed for 5 minutes if there is a strong suspicion of absence seizures. Hyperventilation is not performed in elderly patients and in those with significant vascular disease, since there may be resultant vasospasm and decreased cerebral perfusion.

Sleep deprivation

Sleep deprivation increases the possibility of seeing epileptiform activity in some patients, and also increases the chance of obtaining sleep. Sleep deprivation increases the yield of epileptiform discharges beyond that expected from sleep alone, and therefore is considered a separate physiologic activation method. It is often used for patients in whom routine EEG has not been able to identify interictal epileptiform activity. Sleep deprivation may be a particularly potent activation method in patients with juvenile myoclonic epilepsy. In these patients, the highest yield is in recording most of the EEG after arousal from a brief nap following sleep deprivation.

Normal EEG patterns and variants

Waking and drowsiness

Mu

Mu rhythm is seen in the waking state, and is a negative arch-shaped rhythm of about 8-10 Hz. The potentials are most prominent at C3 and C4. Mu activity is often sharp. Its sharpness and amplitude are increased in the presence of a skull defect over the central region. In drowsiness, the Mu rhythm may be broken up into fragments that can easily be over-interpreted as abnormal epileptiform activity. Mu is very often asymmetrical or unilateral. The absence of Mu activity on one side is not abnormal, unless there is very frequent Mu activity on one side and none on the other side. The key to identification of Mu rhythm is blocking by movement of the contralateral arm. Even contemplating movement can produce this change.

Mu rhythm

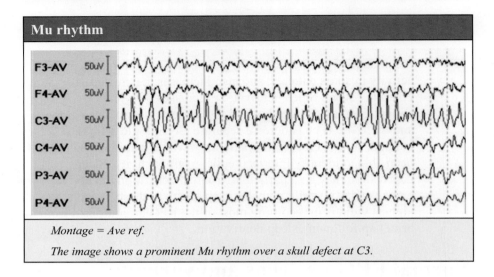

Montage = Ave ref.

The image shows a prominent Mu rhythm over a skull defect at C3.

Third rhythm

This is an alpha range activity recorded in waking and early drowsiness in some patients over the temporal region. This is seen more often in the presence of a skull defect.

Third rhythm

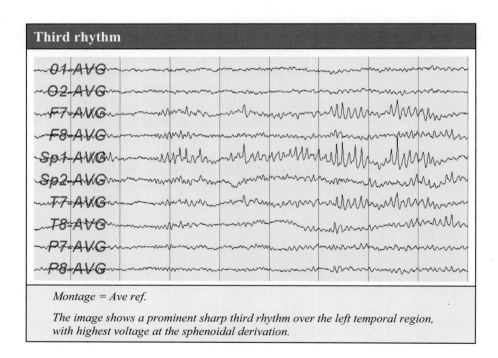

Montage = Ave ref.

The image shows a prominent sharp third rhythm over the left temporal region, with highest voltage at the sphenoidal derivation.

Normal EEG patterns and variants – Rhythms

Rhythm	Description	When present
Mu	Negative arch-shaped rhythmic activity at about 8-10 Hz.	Waking. Attenuated by moving the contralateral arm.
Third rhythm (temporal alpha rhythm)	Alpha range activity in the temporal region	Waking. This is recorded only in some patients. It is not clear what factors influence its appearance, other than skull defect.
Slow alpha variant	Posterior rhythm of 4.5-5 Hz, often notched. A sub-harmonic of the posterior dominant alpha.	Waking. Eyes closed.
Fast alpha variant	Posterior rhythm of 16-20 Hz	Waking. Eyes closed.
SREDA	Periodic sharp activity that evolves into a rhythmic theta pattern, most often parietal in localization.	Older patients in the waking state.
Rhythmic midtemporal theta of drowsiness	Sharply contoured theta trains in the temporal and central regions.	Drowsiness or relaxed wakefulness.
14 & 6 positive spikes	Sharply contoured waves of these frequencies in brief trains. Both frequencies may not be seen, sometimes together. They have a posterior predominance.	Drowsiness and light sleep.

Normal EEG patterns and variants – Transients		
Rhythm	Description	When present
Mu- single transients	Fragments of Mu rhythm	Most likely in drowsiness.
POSTS	Irregular positive waves from the occipital region. These have a similar appearance to lambda waves.	Sleep
Lambda	Positive occipital waves, look like POSTS.	Waking. When viewing a scene or image. Attenuated by eye closure.
Wicket spikes	Sharply contoured waves from the temporal region. These may represent fragments of the *third rhythm*.	Drowsiness and light sleep. More common in older patients.
Rhythmic midtemporal theta of drowsiness	Sharply contoured theta trains in the temporal and central regions.	Drowsiness or relaxed wakefulness
14 & 6 positive spikes	Sharply contoured waves of these frequencies in brief trains. Both frequencies may not be seen.	Drowsiness and light sleep
Phantom spike-waves or 6 Hz spike-and-wave discharges	Low voltage spike-wave complexes that are single or in brief bursts. These have a posterior and mid parietal predominance.	Drowsiness
BSSS (also called SSS and BETS)	Small spike-like potentials in the fronto-temporal regions, typically shifting between the two sides.	Drowsiness and light sleep
Frontal mittens	Mitten-shaped complex formed from the fusion of a sharp alpha or theta transient and a delta wave.	Sleep, especially stage 2

Slow alpha variant

The posterior dominant rhythm in most adults is 8.5-11 Hz. In some patients, there can be a sub-harmonic of the posterior rhythm at 4-5 Hz. The slower frequency is typically notched. The sub-harmonic can be misinterpreted as a slow background in the theta range. Differentiation from slow background can be made by the notched appearance, which is a clue to the faster native background. In addition, the slow alpha variant is attenuated with eye opening. The usual posterior dominant rhythm frequency or the transition between that faster frequency and the slow alpha variant can sometimes be seen elsewhere in the recording. Also, central and anterior activity is of normal frequency composition, whereas most patients with a theta activity background would have abnormal slow activity in these forward regions.

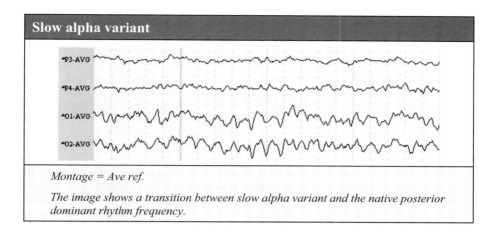

Slow alpha variant

Montage = Ave ref.

The image shows a transition between slow alpha variant and the native posterior dominant rhythm frequency.

Fast alpha variant

In some patients, the posterior dominant rhythm evolves to a harmonic frequency that is twice the native frequency (16-20 Hz). This is a normal variant with no clinical significance.

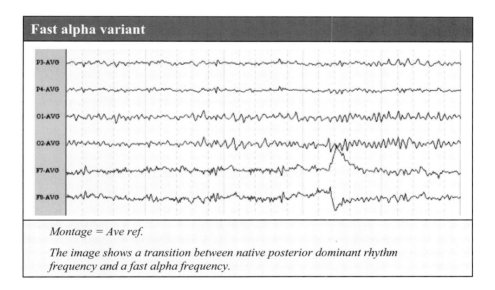

Fast alpha variant

Montage = Ave ref.

The image shows a transition between native posterior dominant rhythm frequency and a fast alpha frequency.

Rhythmic midtemporal theta of drowsiness

Rhythmic midtemporal theta of drowsiness was once called *psychomotor variant*, although this term has been discarded. This pattern consists of trains of sharply contoured notched waves in the theta (6 Hz) range in the temporal region. The pattern may be bilateral, but most often seems to start on one side and within a short time develops on the opposite side.

Rhythmic midtemporal theta of drowsiness

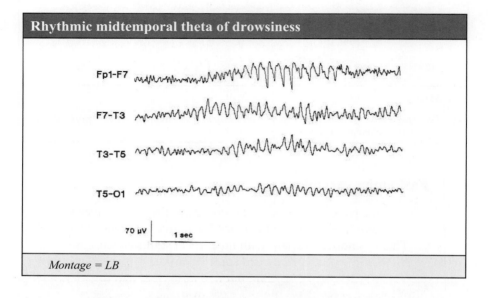

Fp1-F7

F7-T3

T3-T5

T5-O1

70 µV   1 sec

Montage = LB

Rhythmic midtemporal theta of drowsiness is differentiated from seizure activity by presence in drowsiness but not sleep, absence of the evolution in the discharge frequency (which would be typical of seizures) and normal background before and immediately after the discharge.

14 & 6 positive spikes

The 14 & 6 positive spike rhythm is a sharply contoured waveform that is of variable frequency, seen mainly over the temporal regions. At times it is 14 Hz and at others it is 6 Hz, hence the name. However, both frequencies are not necessarily seen in one recording session. The 6 Hz rhythm is most prominent in young children whereas the 14-Hz rhythm predominates in older children. The potentials are seen mainly in drowsiness and light sleep.

14 and 6 Hz positive spikes

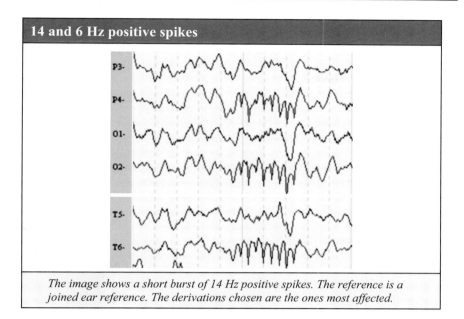

The image shows a short burst of 14 Hz positive spikes. The reference is a joined ear reference. The derivations chosen are the ones most affected.

Historically, there have been some abnormal implications of 14 & 6 Hz positive spike rhythm, but it is now clear that the incidence of these discharges is not different from the general population. When this pattern is seen in an EEG recording, it should be mentioned in the body of the report, but should not be reported as an abnormality.

Lambda waves

Lambda waves are positive waves that are present when viewing a scene or complex image. The waves are blocked by eye closure. These waves resemble POSTs. This pattern is seen in the waking state from the occipital region.

The pattern is completely normal. The lambda waves may be mistaken for occipital spikes, however, their positive polarity and blocking with eye closure make this clearly not epileptiform.

Lambda waves

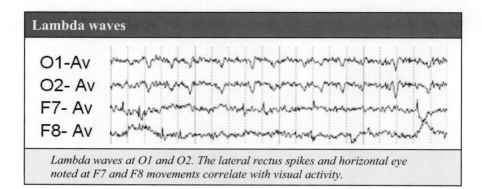

Lambda waves at O1 and O2. The lateral rectus spikes and horizontal eye noted at F7 and F8 movements correlate with visual activity.

Phantom spike-waves

These low voltage 6 Hz spike-and-wave discharges can be single or brief serial and occur typically in drowsiness. The classical benign variant has biposterior predominance, particularly at Pz. They tend to occur mostly in young women.

Phantom spike-waves

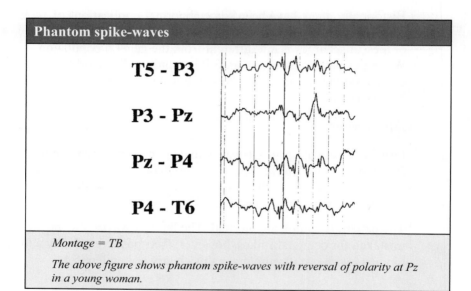

Montage = TB

The above figure shows phantom spike-waves with reversal of polarity at Pz in a young woman.

SREDA

Subclinical rhythmic electrographic discharge of adults (SREDA) is rhythmic sharp activity that appears in some older patients in the awake state. Typically, periodic sharply contoured waves evolve into a rhythmic theta pattern.

Although SREDA resembles an ictal discharge, there is no clinical change during the discharge.

Sleeping

Mittens

Mittens are the result of fusion of a sharply contoured alpha or theta wave with a delta wave in the frontal region. They are only seen in sleep. The slower wave forms the hand of the mitten while the thumb is created by the sharp component.

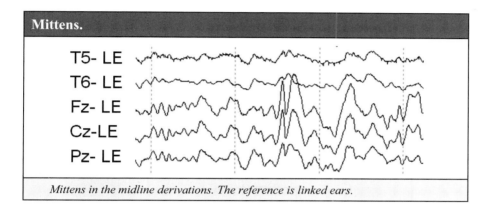

Mittens.

T5- LE

T6- LE

Fz- LE

Cz-LE

Pz- LE

Mittens in the midline derivations. The reference is linked ears.

POSTS

Positive occipital sharp transients of sleep (POSTS), as the name indicates, are positive waves seen most prominently at O1 and O2 during the sleeping stage. They can appear as single waves, or in trains.

POSTS

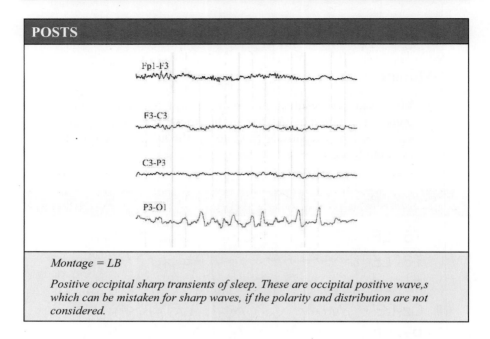

Montage = LB

Positive occipital sharp transients of sleep. These are occipital positive wave,s which can be mistaken for sharp waves, if the polarity and distribution are not considered.

POSTS are differentiated from sharp waves by the positive polarity lack of an following slow wave. POSTS resemble lambda waves, although the latter are seen only in the waking state with the eyes open.

Wicket spikes

Wicket spikes are single or brief trains of sharply contoured waves recorded from the temporal region during drowsiness and light sleep. They are differentiated from epileptiform spikes by their usually symmetrical morphology, the occurrence of similar waves in a rhythm at other times, the absence of a following slow wave, and the normal EEG activity before and after the spikes.

Wicket spikes

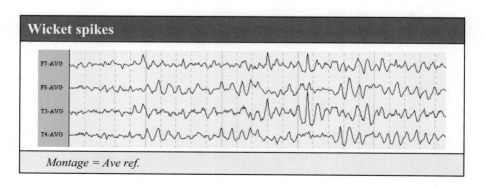

Montage = Ave ref.

BSSS (*benign sporadic sleep spikes*, also called *small sharp spikes* - SSS - and *benign epileptiform transients of sleep* - BETS)

Benign sporadic sleep spikes are very small spike-like potentials that occur in the temporal or frontotemporal regions during drowsiness and light sleep. The duration is less than 50 msec with an amplitude usually less than 50 µV (but they may look larger in long distance derivations). They may be monophasic, biphasic and occasionally polyphasic. They may also have a small after-going slow wave. BSSS are usually differentiated from epileptiform spikes by small amplitude, short duration, tendency to shift from side to side, occasional oblique dipole with negativity in one hemisphere and positivity in another hemisphere, and otherwise normal EEG background. However, the most reliable distinguishing feature is disappearance in deep sleep, while true epileptiform discharges are usually increased in deeper sleep.

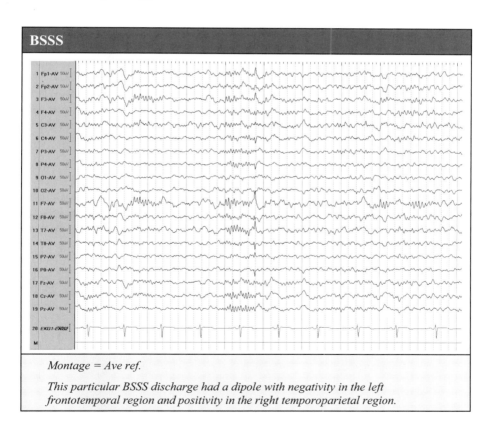

BSSS

Montage = Ave ref.

This particular BSSS discharge had a dipole with negativity in the left frontotemporal region and positivity in the right temporoparietal region.

Non-cerebral potentials

Non-cerebral potentials are always a contaminant, particularly in a hospital setting, and are most likely with recordings made in the ICU. Electrical artifact is especially troublesome when it cannot easily be differentiated from cerebral sharp wave and spike activity. Even non-cerebral slow activity can be confused with slow activity on the EEG.

Eye movement

The eye is electrically charged with the cornea positive relative to the fundus, so any movement of the eye results in potentials that can be recorded from anterior leads. These potentials can occasionally be mistaken for frontal lobe activity. The eyes are almost always moving.

Vertical eye movements

Downward gaze results in the positive cornea moving away from the frontal lobe, so negativity is seen in frontal leads. The reverse is true for upward gaze. Since the eyes move up and down together, the potentials from the two sides are synchronous. Of course, one must remember the possibility of a prosthetic eye, producing unilateral eye movement artifact. Certain vertical eye movements have characteristic patterns, including eye blinks, eye opening, eye closure, eye fluttering.

Eye closure

Eye closure results in Bell's phenomenon, an upward deviation of the eyes. This will be associated with a positive deflection in the frontopolar electrodes. The reason that the tracing returns to baseline is the low frequency filter.

Eye closure

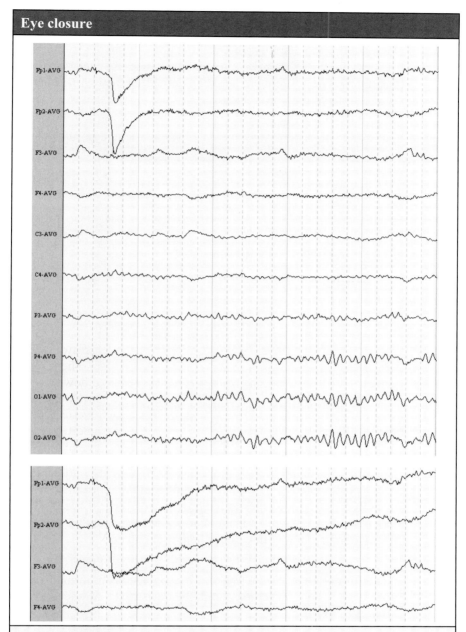

Montage = Ave ref.

With eye closure, there is a positive deflection at Fp1 and Fp2. The rate of return to baseline depends on the setting of the low frequency filter. The lower part of the figure demonstrates the effect of the reducing the low frequency filter setting from 1 Hz to 0.1 Hz Notice the appearance of posterior dominant rhythm in conjunction with eye closure.

Eye blink

An eye blink causes the same positive potential in the frontopolar regions, but the subsequent eye opening causes a negative deflection. The subsequent negative deflection distinguishes an eye blink from mere eye closure.

Eye blinks

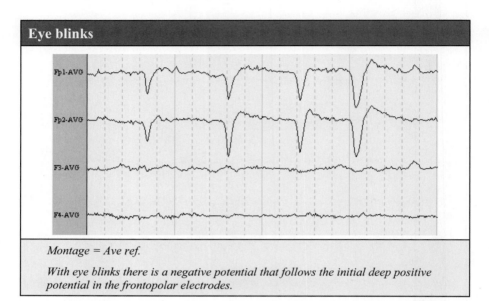

Montage = Ave ref.

With eye blinks there is a negative potential that follows the initial deep positive potential in the frontopolar electrodes.

Eye opening

Eye opening results in a negative potential in the frontopolar electrodes plus alteration in the posterior rhythm. The attenuation of the posterior rhythm with eye opening and reappearance with eye closing are good clues to the presence of vertical eye movements, although the technician should indicate this phenomenon along with other patient movements.

Eye closure results in restoration of the posterior rhythm. The posterior dominant frequency may be slightly faster immediately after closure and, therefore, should be measured a few seconds after eye closure.

Eye opening

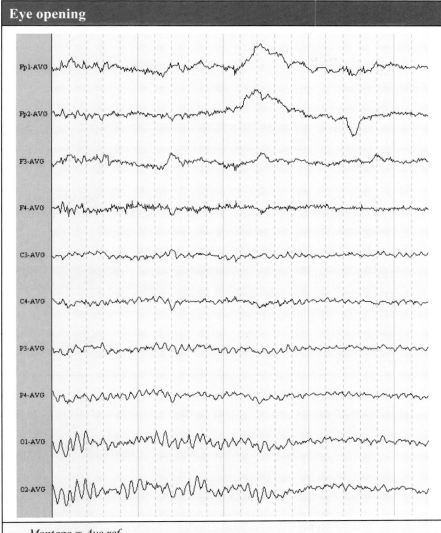

Montage = Ave ref.

With eye opening there is a negative potential in the frontopolar electrodes and attenuation of the posterior dominant rhythm.

Lateral eye movements

Lateral gaze results in the positive cornea moving toward the temple to the side of gaze. For example, left gaze results in positivity at the F7 electrode, whereas there is negativity at the F8 electrode. The differential effect of lateral gaze on the two sides makes for easy identification of this as a non cerebral potential.

Lateral eye movements

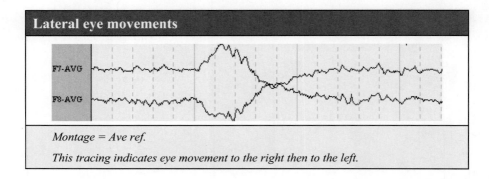

Montage = Ave ref.

This tracing indicates eye movement to the right then to the left.

Lateral eye movements are often associated with lateral rectus spikes. Typically, the spike will be followed by a slower positive potential on the side to which the eyes moved.

Lateral eye movements and lateral rectus spikes

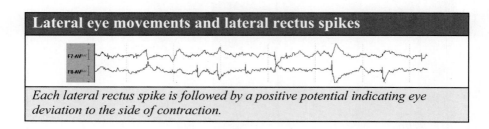

Each lateral rectus spike is followed by a positive potential indicating eye deviation to the side of contraction.

Differentiating eye movement from cerebral potentials is based on some basic guidelines:

- Certain eye movements such as eye blinks have a stereotypic appearance, different from frontal slow activity. In addition, vertical eye movements are generally restricted to, or at least markedly predominant, in the frontopolar electrodes. This has resulted in the principle that slow wave activity restricted to the frontopolar electrodes is eye movement artifact until proven otherwise.
- Pathologic frontal slow activity tends to be associated with a slow background, with activity in the theta and/or delta range. A normal background will suggest that slow activity restricted to the frontal region most likely represents eye movement artifact.
- Patients with marked vertical eye movements will often have prominent lateral eye movements as well, which can be easily recognized.

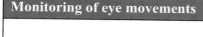

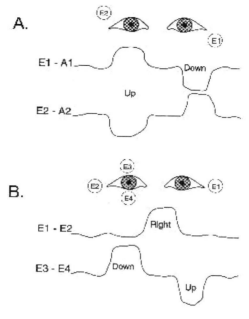

A: Electrodes can be placed above one eye and below the other. Vertical eye movements result in opposite movements of recordings from the two sides. Although this is not shown, horizontal eye movements also result in disparate potentials that can differentiate this from frontal slow activity.

B: A more complex arrangement of leads causes there to be different deflections at the leads with horizontal and vertical gaze. This arrangement is more helpful for documentation of the direction of eye movements than just detection of eye movements.

If there is still doubt, leads are placed around the eye to record eye movements specifically. On the disc are figures and instructions on identification and differentiation of eye movement artifact.

Since the major difficulty will be with vertical eye movements, infraorbital leads are extremely helpful. The figure on page 88 shows the position of infraorbital leads and how they can distinguish cerebral activity, eye movement artifact, and glossokinetic artifact.

Position of infraorbital electrodes

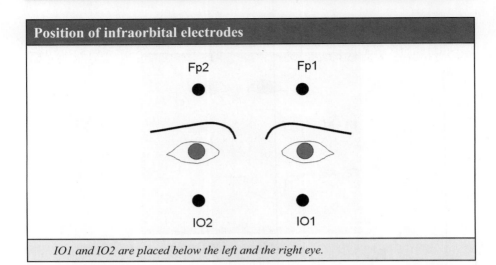

IO1 and IO2 are placed below the left and the right eye.

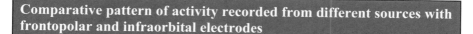

Comparative pattern of activity recorded from different sources with frontopolar and infraorbital electrodes

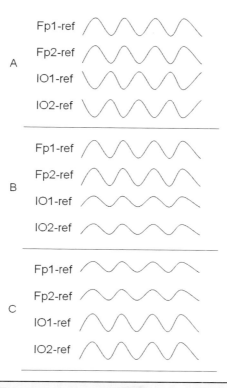

A- *Activity related to vertical eye movements. This will be of opposite polarity in the infraorbital versus the frontopolar electrodes.*

B- *Activity of cerebral origin. This has the same polarity in the infraorbital and frontopolar electrodes, but has lower amplitude in the frontopolar electrodes, which are closer to the frontal cortex.*

C- *Glossokinetic activity arising in the tongue. This has the same polarity in the infraorbital and the frontopolar electrodes, but has higher amplitude in the infraorbital electrodes, which are closer to the tongue.*

Muscle artifact

EMG activity frequently contaminates EEG recordings, and this is prominent when patients are tense, seizing, or have other reasons for increased tone of scalp muscles. EMG is often prominent from the temporal leads. Frontal and occipital leads may also be prominently involved, whereas midline electrodes will usually be least affected. EMG artifact consists of short needle-like spikes that may occur in such frequency that they become confluent and give an appearance that resembles noise. Some guidelines for differentiating EMG from epileptiform spikes are a follows:

- EMG is very fast, much faster than spikes. Activity recorded at the scalp that is shorter than 20 msec is highly unlikely to be epileptiform activity.
- EMG spikes are not followed by a slow wave
- EMG is prominent in the waking state, and disappears with sleep
- EMG spikes recur at a rate that is much faster than would be seen with repetitive spikes.
- EMG is attenuated by asking the patient to relax the jaw, open the mouth, or other similar maneuver.

Muscle artifact

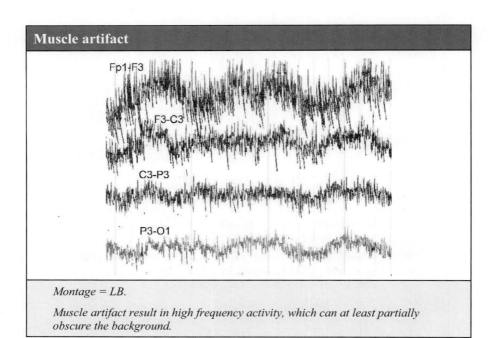

Montage = LB.

Muscle artifact result in high frequency activity, which can at least partially obscure the background.

Occasionally, muscle artifact is more restricted, and may even arise from a single motor unit. Motor unit activity can be noted particularly in the midtemporal region.

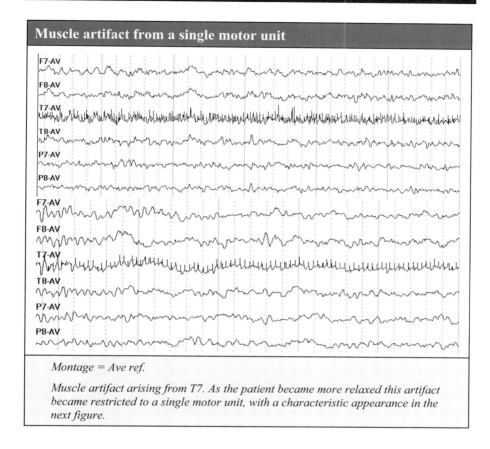

Muscle artifact from a single motor unit

F7-AV

F8-AV

T7-AV

T8-AV

P7-AV

P8-AV

F7-AV

F8-AV

T7-AV

T8-AV

P7-AV

P8-AV

Montage = Ave ref.

Muscle artifact arising from T7. As the patient became more relaxed this artifact became restricted to a single motor unit, with a characteristic appearance in the next figure.

Although muscle artifact can be filtered using the high frequency filter, the unfiltered EEG should always be viewed first. The high frequency filter may distort the appearance of muscle artifact such that it starts to appear cerebral in origin. An example is on page 92.

Effect of high frequency filter on muscle artifact

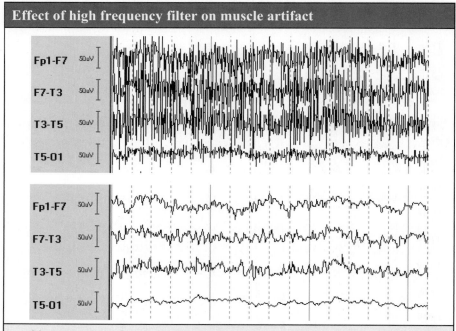

Montage = Ave ref.

The top segment has a high frequency filter setting of 70 Hz, whereas the lower segment has a high frequency setting of 15 Hz. Without looking at the unfiltered EEG, the muscle activity may be misinterpreted as beta activity.

Glossokinetic artifact

The tongue is polarized with the tip negative in comparison to the back. Movement of the tongue is common in the waking state and can occasionally be mistaken for pathologic frontal slow activity. This is potentially even more problematic in a comatose patient who is having tongue movements. Glossokinetic artifact can be differentiated from slow activity in the following ways:

- Glossokinetic artifact usually disappears in drowsiness and light sleep.
- Glossokinetic artifact is associated with activities such as speaking, chewing, swallowing.
- Glossokinetic artifact is often concurrent with EMG artifact of the frontalis and temporalis muscles.

If there is still doubt about identification, then electrodes can be placed below the eyes. The patient is asked to make lingual movements such as "la la la" and the potentials observed are higher in voltage than at the frontopolar electrodes. Cerebral activity will be higher in voltage in the frontopolar electrodes.

Identification of glossokinetic artifact is much better if the technician recognizes the problem and is able to perform these maneuvers.

Combinations of muscle and glossokinetic artifact produce very characteristic patterns. Some are displayed below.

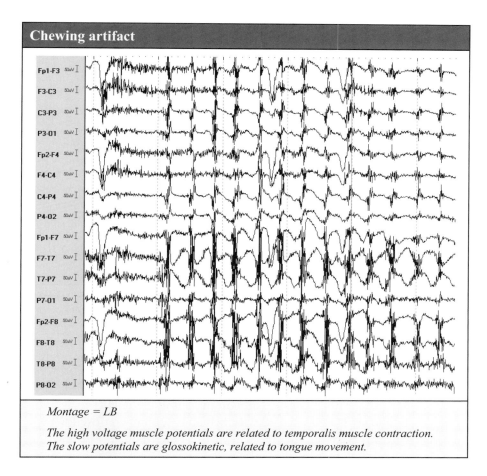

Chewing artifact

Montage = LB

The high voltage muscle potentials are related to temporalis muscle contraction. The slow potentials are glossokinetic, related to tongue movement.

Nonphysiologic electrical artifact

This type of artifact can imitate many abnormal cerebral potentials. We will list only some of the more common nonphysiologic electrical artifacts.

Electrode pop artifact

Electrode pop artifact is due to sudden change in electrode contact. This is associated with a high impedance. This artifact can have the appearance of epileptiform discharges.

Electrode pop artifact

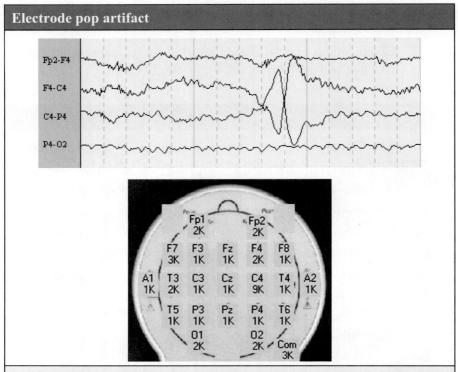

This potential is focal at C4, with no involvement in any other electrode. Electrode impedance measurements obtained at the beginning of the study indicate that C4 impedance was elevated at 9K.

Machine

Machine artifact is especially prominent in the ICU. This is high-frequency stereotyped activity, which is seldom confused with cerebral activity. The frequency can be the frequency of line power, but also can be at faster and slower frequencies, since mechanical devices are not time-locked to line power activity. Most mechanical devices are driven by DC power, although the power comes from AC power through a transformer; therefore, the artifact is the frequency of the motor rather than the frequency of line power. Motors are in ventilators, IV pumps, hospital beds, and other electrical monitoring devices.

60-Hertz

60-Hertz interference is a result of induction from surrounding electronic circuits that are not directly attached to the patient. Movement of current through power lines produces a magnetic field, which is created around the line. This magnetic field causes current to flow in electrode leads by induction, a fundamental property of electronic devices. The induced current flow will reverse at 60-Hz since the magnetic field will also reverse at 60 Hz. Therefore, there is 60 Hz contamination in the electrode leads without any direct connection between the power lines and the EEG leads. This *stray inductance* is a major cause of electrical interference. It is most likely to appear when there is impedance imbalance. It is also most problematic in the ICU environment.

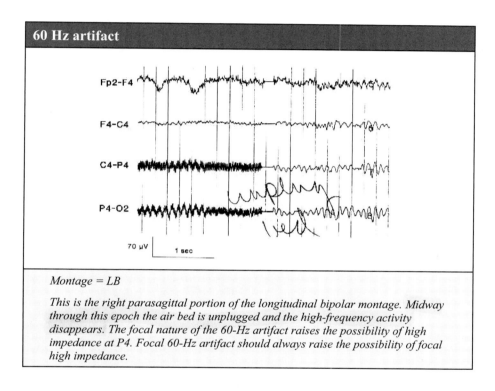

60 Hz artifact

Montage = LB

This is the right parasagittal portion of the longitudinal bipolar montage. Midway through this epoch the air bed is unplugged and the high-frequency activity disappears. The focal nature of the 60-Hz artifact raises the possibility of high impedance at P4. Focal 60-Hz artifact should always raise the possibility of focal high impedance.

How to avoid electrical environmental and machine artifact

Electrical artifact including machine and 60-Hz potentials can be minimized by the following:

- Recording in an electrically quiet environment, certainly not possible for patients in the IC
- Avoidance of ground loops
- Disconnection of all nonessential electronic equipment from the patient
- Minimizing the length of the exposed leads
- Turning off lights and other equipment in proximity to the patient

- Use of differential amplifiers (which is typical with modern equipment) and equal electrode impedances
- Use of the 60-Hz filter, as a last resort

Electrode artifact

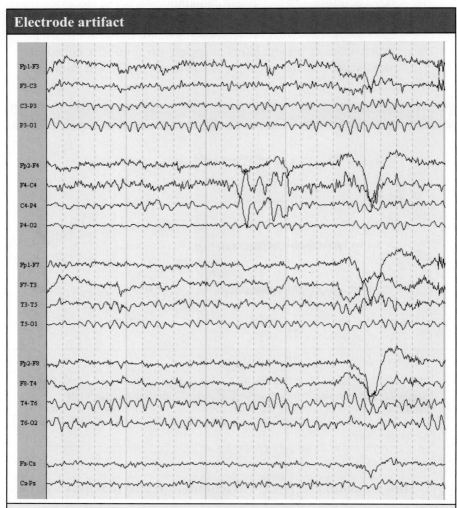

Montage = LB

This example obtained from the same patient above shows sharply contoured slow activity, which has no field, restricted to C4. This makes it likely to be artifactual. It turned out that the technologist had used the 60-Hz filter.

Electrode artifact associated with 60-Hz artifact

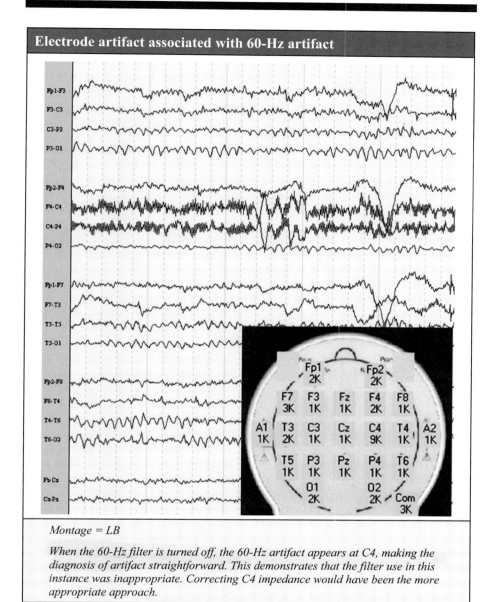

Montage = LB

When the 60-Hz filter is turned off, the 60-Hz artifact appears at C4, making the diagnosis of artifact straightforward. This demonstrates that the filter use in this instance was inappropriate. Correcting C4 impedance would have been the more appropriate approach.

Movement artifact

Movement artifact is due to disturbance of the electrodes and/or leads. Electrode gel is a malleable extension of the electrode, and minor head movement produces little effect on the electrode-gel-scalp attachment. However, movement sufficient to disturb the connection results in charge movement between the electrode and gel and scalp, which is recorded as EEG. Differential amplification does not remove this artifact because the lead artifact is individual.

Movement artifact is also produced by movement of the leads. A small amount of current flows through the electrode leads, and while this current is miniscule compared to most electrical circuits, there is resistance of the leads and capacitance between the leads. This concept of lead circuitry is discussed in more detail on the disc. Movement of the leads results in disturbance of the capacitance. The built-up charge can dissipate with loss of the capacitance, and this too is recorded as EEG.

Movement artifact related to head motion with hyperventilation

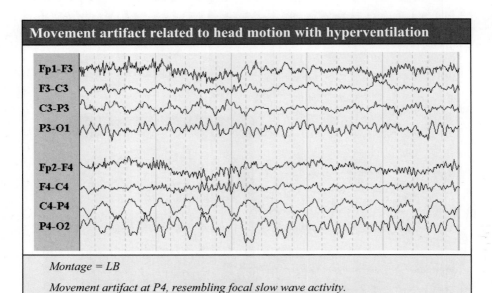

Montage = LB

Movement artifact at P4, resembling focal slow wave activity.

Chapter 6.
Abnormal EEG:
Non-epileptiform
abnormalities

Types of Abnormalities

Abnormal EEG activity includes ictal, interictal epileptiform, and non-epileptiform abnormalities. Non-epileptiform abnormalities will be discussed first. Ictal and interictal epileptiform abnormalities are discussed in the subsequent chapter.

The non-epileptiform abnormalities may include:

- Focal slow activity
- Generalized asynchronous slow activity
- Generalized or regional bisynchronous slow activity
- Focal attenuation
- Generalized attenuation
- Focal and generalized increase in activity
- Periodic discharges
- Other abnormal activity (alpha, theta, and spindle coma patterns, etc.)

Slow activity

Focal slow activity

Focal slow activity usually indicates a focal subcortical structural lesion. The slow activity typically has an irregular, polymorphic appearance, hence the name *polymorphic delta activity* (PDA). In general, the area of the slow activity is overlying the location of the structural lesion, but the anatomic correlation is not always exact.

Focal and generalized slow activity

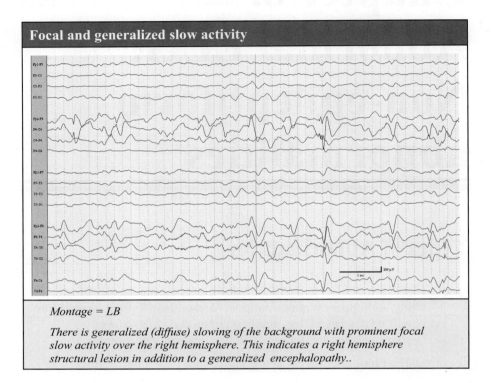

Montage = LB

There is generalized (diffuse) slowing of the background with prominent focal slow activity over the right hemisphere. This indicates a right hemisphere structural lesion in addition to a generalized encephalopathy..

The differential diagnosis of focal irregular slow activity is large, with some of the possibilities including:

- Tumor
- Stroke – ischemic or hemorrhagic
- Infection – abscess or encephalitis
- Trauma – contusion or hematoma
- Epileptic focus producing irregular focal slowing in the absence of a structural lesion
- Migraine producing transient focal slowing
- Postictal slowing after a focal seizure

Unfortunately, one cannot usually be definite about the etiology of the slow activity from the appearance. While additional historical information may help the analysis, the diagnosis of focal structural lesions rests largely with imaging studies.

One form of focal slow activity, *temporal intermittent rhythmic delta activity* (TIRDA), has a strong association with seizure activity.

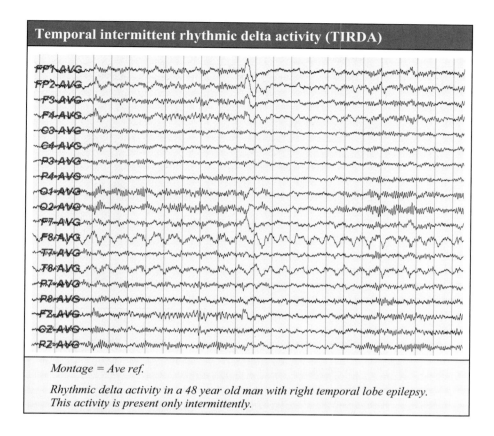

Temporal intermittent rhythmic delta activity (TIRDA)

Montage = Ave ref.

Rhythmic delta activity in a 48 year old man with right temporal lobe epilepsy. This activity is present only intermittently.

Generalized asynchronous slow activity

Generalized asynchronous slow activity is extremely nonspecific. It can be predominantly in the theta or delta range. It usually indicates encephalopathy. Slow activity in the theta range indicates mild encephalopathy whereas slow activity in the delta range means more severe encephalopathy.

Presence of expected normal background for age influences the interpretation of the slow activity, since slow activity is normally present in drowsiness and sleep at all ages and in the awake state in children. In these situations, there should be caution in interpretation of slow activity - we should only read it as abnormal if the pattern is inconsistent with any normal stage of the sleep-wake cycle.

Generalized asynchronous slow activity

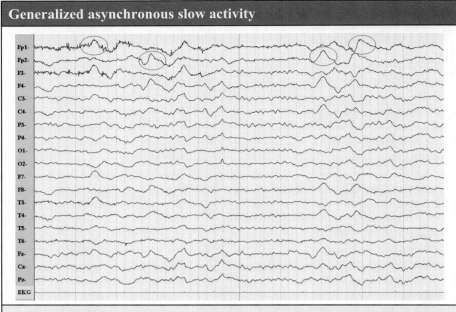

Montage = Ref.

The EEG shows mostly asynchronous generalized slow activity. Specific delta waves seen on one side and not the other are circled. The patient is 74 year old woman with anoxic brain injury.

Generalized asynchronous slow activity

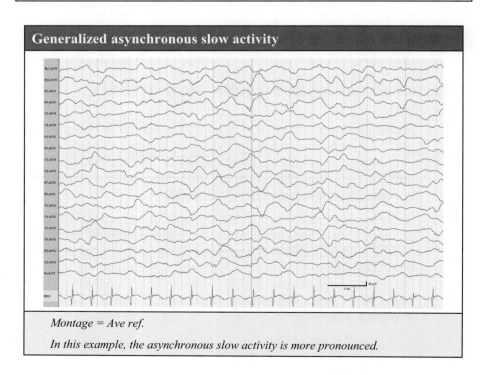

Montage = Ave ref.

In this example, the asynchronous slow activity is more pronounced.

Generalized or regional bisynchronous slow activity

Bisynchronous slow activity can be generalized or regional. Even when it is generalized it usually predominates in one region of the brain. This type of activity is often, but not always, rhythmic and intermittent. The most important is *frontal intermittent rhythmic delta activity* (FIRDA) and *occipital intermittent rhythmic delta activity* (OIRDA).

Frontal intermittent rhythmic delta activity

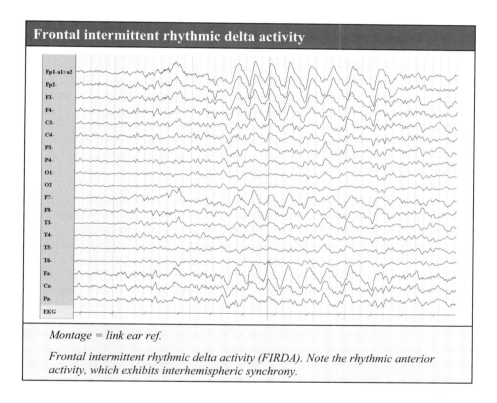

Montage = link ear ref.

Frontal intermittent rhythmic delta activity (FIRDA). Note the rhythmic anterior activity, which exhibits interhemispheric synchrony.

FIRDA is rhythmic activity in the delta range that is synchronous on the two sides. This is either limited to the frontal region or generalized with frontal predominance. The frequency is most often about 2.5-3 Hz. FIRDA can be seen in a variety of conditions, but generally is interpreted as an abnormal interaction between the cerebral cortex and the thalamus. The differential diagnosis includes:

- Metabolic encephalopathies
- Degenerative disorders and other conditions affecting cortical and subcortical gray matter

- Deep midline tumors
- Normal- FIRDA is normal in drowsiness and with hyperventilation at any age and in waking in children

Children have intermittent rhythmic delta activity that tends to be centered over the occipital region rather than the frontal region, hence *occipital intermittent rhythmic delta activity* (OIRDA). Some neurophysiologists prefer the term PIRDA for posterior-IRDA, finding the acronym OIRDA hard to pronounce. The clinical implications of OIRDA in children was considered identical to FIRDA in adults. However, OIRDA was reported to be associated with epilepsy in children, particularly generalized epilepsy. There may be subtle spikes embedded in the occipital rhythmic activity in children with childhood absence epilepsy. Generalized absence and generalized tonic-clonic seizures were more likely in children with OIRDA than in control subjects.

Occipital intermittent rhythmic delta activity

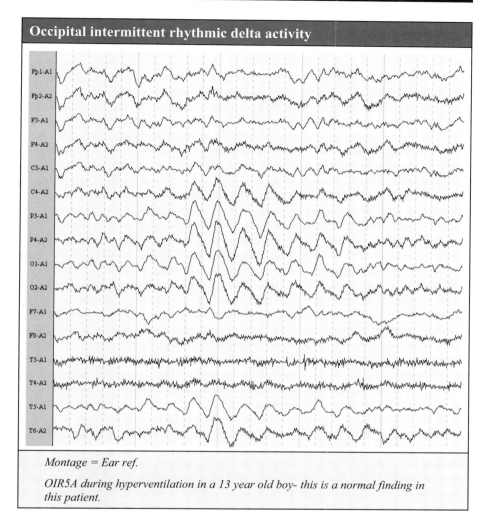

Montage = Ear ref.

OIR5A during hyperventilation in a 13 year old boy- this is a normal finding in this patient.

Attenuation/ suppression

Focal attenuation

The term *attenuation* indicates decreased amplitude of one type of activity (such as activity at a certain frequency) or of all activity. Focal attenuation usually indicates a focal cortical lesion (such as infarct or tumor) or dysfunction (from ischemia or post-ictal effect), but may also result from an increased distance between the cortex and the recording electrode, such as may be seen from scalp edema, subdural hematoma, and occasionally from dural-based tumors, such as meningiomas.

Focal attenuation of posterior alpha rhythm

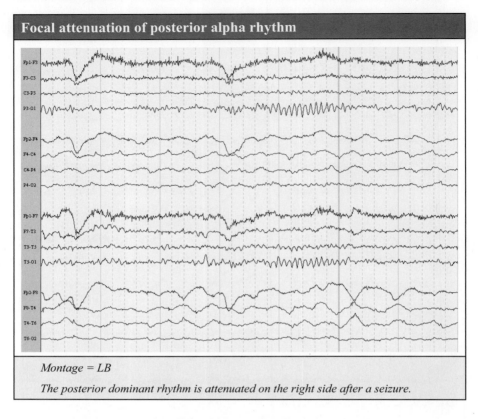

Montage = LB

The posterior dominant rhythm is attenuated on the right side after a seizure.

Generalized attenuation/suppression

The term *suppression* is a more severe attenuation, and is usually used to indicate complete or almost complete disappearance of EEG activity. Generalized attenuation or suppression of the background can happen for three reasons:

- Decreased synchronicity of cortical activity
- Decreased cortical activity
- Excessive fluid or tissue overlying the cortex

Decreased synchronicity of cortical activity may occur in an awake, alert state, and is rarely abnormal; it is often seen in anxious individuals. One normal variant seen in a small proportion of adults is a low voltage background that looks suppressed. However, a low voltage EEG would be abnormal in children and adolescents.

Attenuated EEG as a normal variant

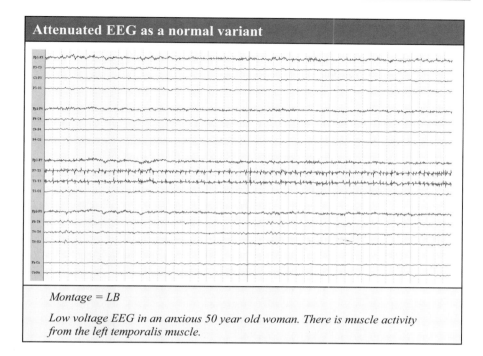

Montage = LB

Low voltage EEG in an anxious 50 year old woman. There is muscle activity from the left temporalis muscle.

Generalized decreased cortical activity can occur with generalized cortical injury or transient dysfunction. Examples of cortical injury include generalized suppression as a sequela of *hypoxic-ischemic encephalopathy* (HIE) or generalized suppression from conditions such as advanced Huntington's disease. Examples of transient dysfunction include generalized suppression from drug-induced coma or postictal state after a generalized tonic-clonic seizure.

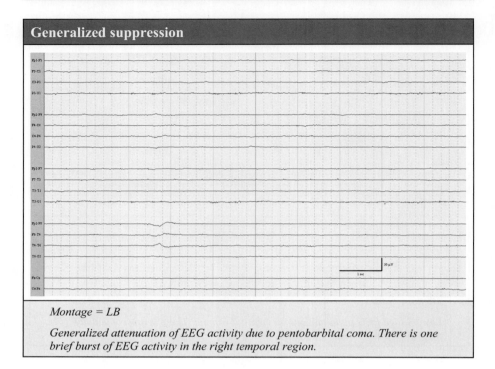

Montage = LB

Generalized attenuation of EEG activity due to pentobarbital coma. There is one brief burst of EEG activity in the right temporal region.

Excessive fluid or tissue overlying the cortex is more likely to produce focal rather than generalized attenuation. Examples include subdural hematoma or scalp edema. With subdural hematoma, the attenuation is most pronounced with bipolar recordings: there is cortical activity, but the conducting ability of the subdural fluid results in cancellation of potential differences and attenuates the recorded potential at the scalp. The same shunting of potential differences may occur with electrode gel smear on the scalp (often called salt bridge or electrical bridge).

Isoelectric EEG

Isoelectric EEG represents absence of electrocerebral activity. The definition of an isoelectric EEG is one with no cerebral activity over 2 µV. The technical requirements of an isoelectric EEG are:

- Electrodes >10 cm apart
- Electrode impedance between 100 Ω and 6000 Ω
- Hypothermia, drug intoxication, shock must be excluded
- Record should be > 30 min long at a sensitivity of 2 µV/mm

- • Physiological monitoring must include EKG. Other physiological monitoring such as respiration and EMG is very helpful.

The background will look totally flat at a sensitivity of 7 μV/mm. However, at a sensitivity of 2 μV/mm, the recording is never perfectly flat, and if it appears to be, either the gain needs to be increased or there has to be an electrical problem in the recording system. The residual activity in the EEG should be proven to be of artifactual origin. In fact, artifacts are a major problem in interpretation. The artifact most commonly encountered is EKG artifact, which may take on a variable appearance at the scalp. Demonstrating perfect correlation with EKG is usually sufficient to prove the activity is not cerebral. The same is true for artifact due to respiration. However, a variety of rhythmic activity can be due to machine artifact, movement artifact, or muscle artifact. The EEG technologist may need to disconnect nonessential equipment, reposition the patient, pad respirator tubes with towels, or move electrodes. The patient may need to be paralyzed if the EEG is contaminated with muscle artifact.

ECS not necessarily equivalent to brain death. An isoelectric EEG indicates neocortical death and is supportive of the diagnosis of brain death in conjunction with the appropriate exam findings, if performed in accordance with accepted technical guidelines. Details of brain death criteria are discussed on the disc.

Focal increase in EEG activity

Focal increase in EEG activity is most often the result of a skull defect. Since the skull filters fast activity, the presence of a defect is most likely to cause increased fast beta activity, as well as increased sharpness of EEG activity. Sharpness represents a higher frequency component of EEG activity, indicating altered frequency attenuation without the bone.

Specific rhythms can become more prominent with skull defects in specific regions. For example, if the skull defect is over the central region, Mu activity may be exaggerated, and if the skull defect is over the temporal region, a third rhythm could become more prominent. The EEG activity over skull defects in these areas is often referred to as a *breach rhythm*. It is not clear that this should necessarily be considered an abnormality. It is rather an expected effect of a skull defect.

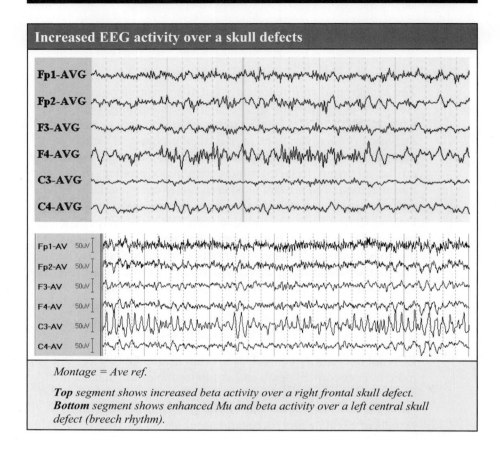

Increased EEG activity over a skull defects

Montage = Ave ref.

Top *segment shows increased beta activity over a right frontal skull defect.*
Bottom *segment shows enhanced Mu and beta activity over a left central skull defect (breech rhythm).*

Generalized increase in EEG activity

Excessive fast activity

Excessive fast activity is most commonly seen in patients receiving sedatives such as barbiturates or benzodiazepines. Chloral hydrate usually produces less excessive beta activity.

EMG activity from scalp muscles can appear as fast activity if its voltage is low, and when the high frequency filter is used. This can be differentiated from cerebral fast activity by asking the patient to relax and open the mouth.

Excessive beta should be interpreted as a minor abnormality, and the report should mention that a common cause is sedative medication. The neurophysiologists should not make this absolute determination without full knowledge of the patient, of course.

Excessive slow activity

This is discussed with slow activity, on the previous pages.

Periodic patterns

Periodic discharges are repeated discharges with other intervening activity in between the discharges. They can be classified as *lateralized* or *generalized/bilateral periodic* discharges. Lateralized periodic discharges are often called *periodic lateralized epileptiform discharges* (PLEDs) even if the individual waveforms are not epileptiform. Generalized periodic discharges can be classified as *short interval* and *long interval* periodic discharges. Burst-suppression could also be considered a periodic pattern.

Periodic lateralized epileptiform discharges (PLEDs)

PLEDs are periodic discharges that are lateralized to one hemisphere. This will include discharges that are focal, as well as others that affect one whole hemisphere. Some lesser involvement of the other hemisphere is acceptable under the description of lateralized. Even though the term PLEDs excludes bihemispheric synchronous periodic discharges, PLEDs can occur independently in the two hemispheres, in which case they are termed *biPLEDs*.

PLEDs are usually high in amplitude, at 100-300 µV. Lower voltage PLEDs can be difficult to identify in the background. The discharge may be simple or complex, with additional sharp and slow components superimposed on the waveform. In general, PLEDs are diagnosed only if they are present throughout the routine 20 minute EEG recording.

Periodic lateralized epileptiform discharges

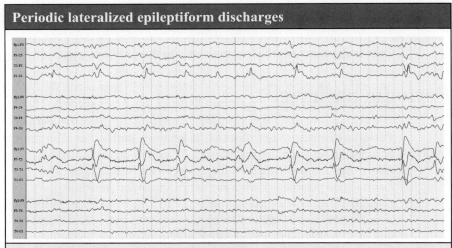

Montage = LB

Examples of PLEDs seen from the left hemisphere. There is a slight reflection of PLEDs in the right hemisphere, which is not unusual.

The patient developed confusion, aphasia, and witnessed focal motor seizure activity of the right arm and face 10 days after a left carotid endarterectomy, and was found to have a hyperperfusion syndrome.

PLEDs are most often the result of acute structural lesion, such as stroke, acute infection or rapidly growing brain tumor (for example glioblastoma multiforme). However, PLEDs can also occur in patients with acute metabolic disturbance who also have a chronic structural lesion (especially in the setting of alcohol withdrawal). PLEDs can also occur in the setting of chronic epilepsy. Therefore PLEDs are not specific for a particular diagnosis. PLEDs in the temporal or frontotemporal area can be a sign of herpes encephalitis.

The majority of patients with PLEDs have clinical seizures. However, there is a controversy over whether PLEDs themselves are ictal. The prevailing opinion is that PLEDs are not ictal, because more typical rhythmic ictal discharges are sometimes recorded in patients with PLEDs. However, there are patients with PLEDs who have myoclonic jerks synchronous with the discharges, suggesting that they may be ictal in some instances.

PLEDS are more likely to be ictal if they have any of the following features:

- Fast rhythmic activity with the periodic complexes
- Short interval between discharges
- Absence of background in between discharges

Generalized periodic discharges

Generalized periodic discharges may be prevalent in one part of the brain, usually anteriorly. They are often classified as short interval or long interval periodic discharges. Short interval periodic discharges have a periodicity of 0.5-3 per second. They are more common and less specific than long interval discharges. The main underlying conditions include:

- Metabolic disturbances (e.g. triphasic waves with hepatic encephalopathy)
- Anoxic injury
- Toxic encephalopathy
- Creutzfeld-Jakob disease
- Nonconvulsive status epilepticus

Clinical correlation is always required. In Creutzfeld-Jakob disease, the majority of patients will develop periodic discharges in the first 3 months of the disease.

Generalized periodic discharges (CJD)

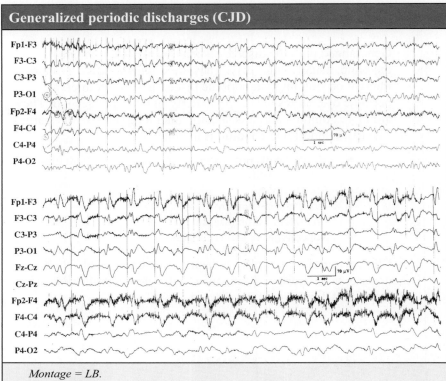

Montage = LB.

*69 year old patient with Creutzfeld-Jakob disease. **Top** tracing showed only subtle periodic discharges that are easy to miss. **Bottom** tracing obtained 2 weeks later showed very clear periodic discharges with a periodicity of 1.2 per second (Courtesy of Dr Ivo Drury).*

Long-term periodic discharges have intervals of at least 4 seconds between discharges. They are more specific with respect to etiology, particularly when the clinical history is incorporated. Associated conditions include:

- Some toxic encephalopathies (e.g. baclofen, PCP, ketamine)
- Anoxic injury
- Subacute sclerosing panencephalitis (SSPE)

SSPE is suggested by long interval periodic discharges in the setting of a child with dementia and myoclonic jerks. In this condition, the interval between complexes becomes progressively shorter with disease progression.

Long interval generalized periodic discharges (SSPE)

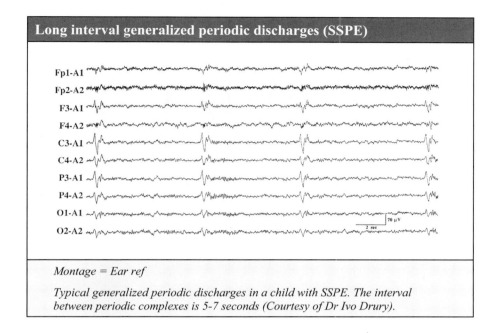

Montage = Ear ref

Typical generalized periodic discharges in a child with SSPE. The interval between periodic complexes is 5-7 seconds (Courtesy of Dr Ivo Drury).

Burst-suppression pattern

The *burst-suppression pattern* is sometimes called the *suppression-burst pattern* when the duration of the suppression is greater than the duration of the burst. This pattern is seen mainly in patients with severe encephalopathy although the pattern is not specific for any particular etiology. The most common causes are:

- Hypoxic-ischemic encephalopathy
- Barbiturate coma.

The burst-suppression pattern consists of epochs of relative flattening of the background (the suppression) alternating with epochs of mixed frequency EEG activity (the bursts). The bursts usually have a polymorphic appearance, but may contain high voltage epileptiform activity in some patients who are placed in barbiturate coma for refractory status epilepticus.

Burst-suppression patterns can look similar even though the clinical correlation is very different. In fact, this pattern resembles the discontinuous pattern of a normal 19-week conceptional age child, suggesting that the burst-suppression pattern may represent a primitive pattern of neuronal activity.

With drug induced coma, the deeper the coma, the shorter the bursts and the longer the periods of suppression. Eventually complete suppression is reached.

Burst-suppression pattern

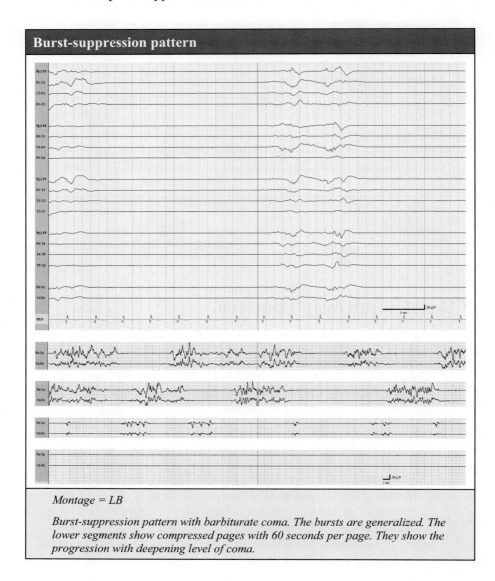

Montage = LB

Burst-suppression pattern with barbiturate coma. The bursts are generalized. The lower segments show compressed pages with 60 seconds per page. They show the progression with deepening level of coma.

When seen in hypoxic-ischemic encephalopathy, the burst-suppression pattern is indicative of a poor prognosis for neurological recovery. In fact, any periodic pattern is a poor prognostic indicator in this clinical setting.

Burst-suppression pattern

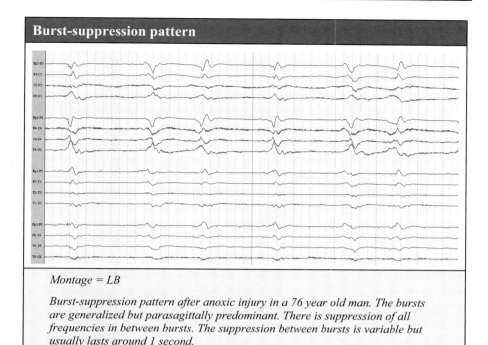

Montage = LB

Burst-suppression pattern after anoxic injury in a 76 year old man. The bursts are generalized but parasagittally predominant. There is suppression of all frequencies in between bursts. The suppression between bursts is variable but usually lasts around 1 second.

Other non-epileptiform abnormalities

This heterogeneous category includes a number of abnormalities that are difficult to put together. The most important are alpha coma, theta coma, and spindle coma. All these coma patterns are nonspecific with respect to etiology or prognosis. Typically, the prognosis is poor if the etiology is hypoxic-ischemic. The presence of reactivity is indicative of a more favorable prognosis.

Alpha coma can have two main patterns: one that is usually associated with generalized cerebral insult/dysfunction, and another that occurs with pontine lesions. In generalized cerebral dysfunction, the alpha activity tends to have a generalized, sometimes frontally dominant distribution and to be unreactive to stimulation. In pontine lesions, alpha activity tends to be posteriorly dominant and is often reactive to eye opening and closure.

Alpha coma pattern

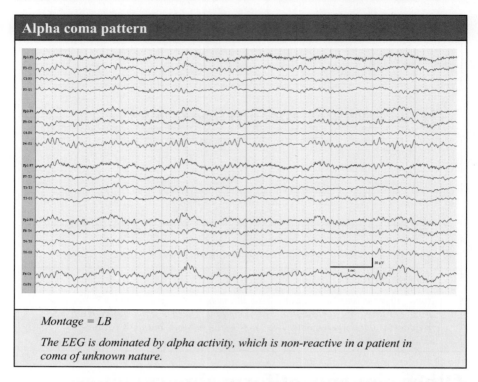

Montage = LB

The EEG is dominated by alpha activity, which is non-reactive in a patient in coma of unknown nature.

Spindle coma pattern

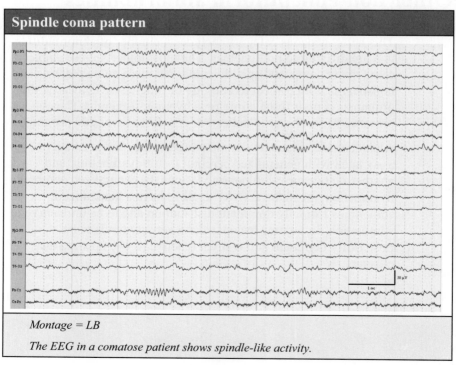

Montage = LB

The EEG in a comatose patient shows spindle-like activity.

EEG patterns with selected specific conditions

Herpes simplex encephalitis (HSE)

HSE usually shows PLEDs at some point during the disease. PLEDs usually start after the second day of symptoms, and last no more than a few days to 2 weeks. They may be unilateral or bilateral, but are not synchronous from the two hemispheres. The PLEDs are sharply contoured waves repeating every 1 – 2.5 seconds. The duration of each wave is at least 50 ms. PLEDS recorded from one temporal region are the most distinctive for HSE.

Neonatal HSE is characterized by necrosis that is not confined to the temporal region, and is often not most prominent there. These patients may have multifocal PLEDs, and the EEG may show attenuation of the background with poor organization and slow activity in the delta range.

Stroke

Stroke commonly produces focal slow activity over the region of infarction or hemorrhage, although with extensive cortical involvement, focal or lateralized attenuation of EEG activity may be the predominant finding. PLEDs may also be seen. In fact, stroke is the most common cause of PLEDs. This EEG pattern cannot, by itself, differentiate between stroke and other acute or rapidly evolving structural lesions such as tumors and encephalitis.

Hemorrhage and infarction can produce similar appearance on the EEG, although there may be more sharp activity with hemorrhage – this is not a clinically important differentiating feature. Subarachnoid hemorrhage can have a spectrum of abnormality, which is usually not localized, unlike with intraparenchymal hemorrhage or infarction. There can be slowing of background rhythms, attenuation, or even the appearance of the burst-suppression pattern.

Acute stroke with attenuation

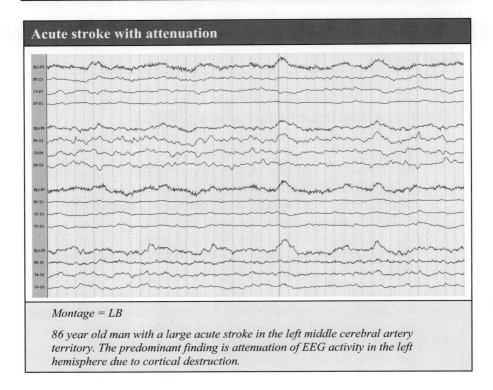

Montage = LB

86 year old man with a large acute stroke in the left middle cerebral artery territory. The predominant finding is attenuation of EEG activity in the left hemisphere due to cortical destruction.

Alzheimer's disease (AD)

The EEG is seldom ordered in patients with suspected AD. It is usually ordered to look for epileptiform activity in patients with dementia who have had seizure, syncope, or some other spell. In addition, patients with rapidly progressive dementia may have an EEG ordered to look for periodic discharges that could be supportive of prion disease.

Patients with AD usually have slowing of the waking posterior rhythm. They will occasionally have a normal background, especially early in the course of the disease. Therefore, a normal EEG is not evidence against AD unless the dementia appears severe in the presence of a normal background, in which case psychological causes for memory and cognitive dysfunction should be considered. Late in the course of the disease, patients may develop generalized asynchronous and synchronous slow activity. AD is a risk factor for epilepsy, and seizures and epileptiform activity do develop in a minority of patients.

Creutzfeldt-Jakob disease (CJD)

CJD shows a typical periodic pattern at some point in the disease process, but not at all times in the disease. These periodic discharges usually appear within 3 months of onset of symptoms. The abnormality is a sharp wave or sharply contoured slow wave with a periodicity of 0.5-2/sec. The discharges are maximal in the anterior regions and may even occasionally be unilateral. Late in the course of the disease, the discharges are more prominent posteriorly and when so, are commonly associated with blindness. The discharges may or may not be temporally locked to the myoclonus.

The discharges are superimposed on an abnormal background characterized by low-voltage slowing in the theta and delta range. The periodic complexes abate in sleep.

Early in the course, the periodic complexes may not be seen and the only finding may be focal or generalized slow activity. About 10-15% of patients may not show periodic patterns during their course.

Creutzfeldt-Jakob disease

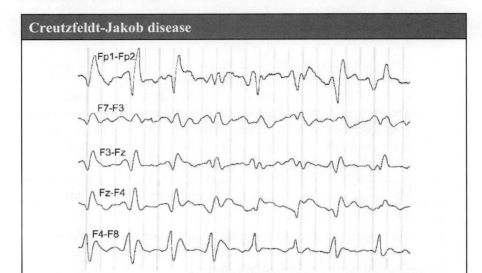

Montage = TB

Periodic pattern typical of CJD. This pattern is not specific for this diagnosis, but in the appropriate clinical situation is supportive of the diagnosis. Note that this pattern is not seen at all stages.

Hypoxic-ischemic encephalopathy (HIE)

Hypoxic-ischemic encephalopathy is also called *anoxic encephalopathy*, since the most common cause is cardiac arrest where there is loss of oxygenation and/or reduced blood flow to the brain.

The EEG can have different appearances including:

- Generalized asynchronous and/or bisynchronous slow activity
- Generalized attenuation
- Alpha coma
- Theta coma
- Spindle coma
- Periodic discharges
- Burst-suppression
- Generalized suppression

Periodic discharges are highly variable in appearance and periodicity. They may be synchronous or independent from the two hemispheres. The repetitive discharges are not considered epileptiform by most neurophysiologists. The discharges can look like PLEDs except for the synchronous appearance from the two hemispheres. Myoclonus may or may not be synchronous with the discharges.

The burst-suppression pattern is commonly seen in HIE and is characterized by bursts of slow waves in the theta and delta range sometimes with sharp or fast activity superimposed on the slow activity. The bursts vary greatly in duration, as does the interburst suppression.

Suppression of the background is a more extreme abnormality. The appearance is similar to the suppressed portion of the burst-suppression pattern.

HIE usually has a particularly poor prognosis in the presence of periodic discharges, burst suppression or suppression.

Chapter 7.
Abnormal EEG:
The EEG in Epilepsy

Role in Diagnosis and Management

The EEG provides support for the clinical diagnosis of epilepsy but should generally not be the basis for that diagnosis in the absence of clinical information.

The EEG has a role in all the following

- Help diagnose epilepsy
- Help diagnose status epilepticus
- Help classify the epilepsy and epileptic syndrome
- Localization of the epileptogenic zone
- Prediction of seizure recurrence after a first unprovoked seizure or after antiepileptic drug withdrawal
- Following response to therapy in idiopathic generalized epilepsy with absence seizures
- Infrequently, providing evidence for the etiology of epilepsy

Patients with idiopathic generalized epilepsy with absence seizures show decreased epileptiform discharges with improvement in seizure control. This correlation between interictal and ictal manifestation is not seen in most other epilepsies.

The EEG is usually not specific to etiology, although differentiation between generalized and focal discharges can help differentiate between idiopathic and symptomatic epilepsies.

Steps in the EEG Analysis in Patients with Suspected Epilepsy

When discharges are found that are suspicious for interictal or ictal activity in epilepsy, there are a sequence of questions that should be asked to assist clinical interpretation.

- Is the discharge cerebral or artifactual?
- If the discharge is cerebral, is it normal or abnormal?
- If the discharge is abnormal, is it epileptiform?
- If the discharge is epileptiform, is it focal or generalized?
- If the discharge is focal, what is the field of the discharge?

Discharges Associated with Epilepsy

In the routine 20 to 30 minute EEG, it is most likely that only interictal abnormalities will be seen. These are the abnormalities most often sought in routine EEGs in epilepsy. Interictal abnormalities that are specific for epilepsy are termed *epileptiform*. It is generally suggested that the term *epileptiform* be reserved for interictal discharges associated with epilepsy, while ictal EEG findings are termed *seizure patterns* or *ictal patterns*. Seizure patterns are infrequently seen in the routine EEG. One notable exception is the ictal discharges of absence seizures. Absence seizures are usually precipitated with hyperventilation in the untreated child with absence epilepsy.

Epileptiform discharges

The most common epileptiform discharges are spikes and sharp waves and combinations of these with slow waves. By definition, spikes are shorter than 70 ms whereas sharp waves are 70-100 ms in duration.

The spectrum of epileptiform discharges includes:

- Spikes
- Sharp waves
- Spike-and-wave complexes
- Slow spike-and-wave complexes
- Sharp-and-slow-wave complexes
- Multiple-spike complexes (or polyspike complexes)
- Multiple-spike-and-slow-wave complexes (or polyspike-and-slow-wave complexes)

- Multiple-sharp-wave complexes
- Multiple-sharp-and-slow-wave complexes

Many EEG waves have a sharp appearance, but they are only called spikes or sharp waves if they satisfy a number of features including:

- A relatively high voltage compared to the background
- An asymmetric appearance typically with a shorter first half and a longer and higher-voltage second half
- A biphasic or polyphasic morphology
- And after-going slow wave

Spikes and sharp waves should be differentiated from surrounding rhythmic activity by more than just a higher voltage sharp component. The great majority of sharp waves and spikes are surface negative. They generally have a field that includes more than one electrode. They should be different from what is expected as physiologic activity in the particular field and state of alertness. Not all the above features have to be present; however, the more features present, the more confident one can be of the epileptiform nature of the activity.

Epileptiform discharges

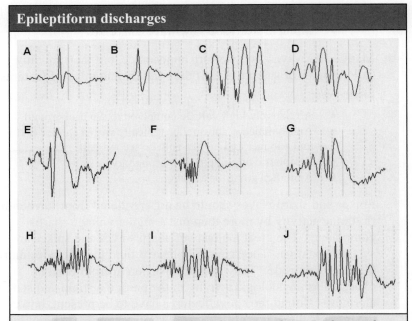

*A- spike; **B**- sharp wave; **C**- spike-and-wave complexes; **D**- sharp-and-slow-wave complexes; **E**- slow-spike-and-wave complex; **F**- polyspike-and-wave complex; **G**- multiple-sharp-and-slow-wave complex; **H**-polyspike complex; **I&J**- multiple sharp wave complexes. Even though spikes and sharp waves usually have after-going slow waves, the term spike-and-wave complex is usually reserved for the situation where the slow wave is very prominent, higher in voltage than the spike. The interval between vertical lines represents 200 msec.*

Ictal versus interictal epileptiform discharges

Ictal discharges are usually not repetition of interictal discharges and will typically have an appearance different from multiple interictal discharges. One exception to this statement is generalized absence seizures, for which the distinction between interictal and ictal discharges is not always clear-cut. For example, in patients with generalized absence seizures it has been demonstrated that a subtle alteration of responsiveness occurs even with a single spike-and-wave discharge. On the other hand, generalized spike-and-wave discharges that are shorter than 3 seconds in duration are typically not noticed by family members, particularly in the absence of motor accompaniments. Therefore, for practical purposes, one could state that bursts of generalized spike-and-wave discharges are ictal if they last more than 3 seconds, or if they are associated with clear clinical changes.

Another pattern that can be ictal or "interictal" is paroxysmal fast activity noted in patients with symptomatic generalized epilepsy, particularly those with Lennox-Gastaut syndrome. In these patients, the paroxysmal fast activity (or generalized polyspike activity) can be associated with generalized tonic seizures or could be totally asymptomatic. Occasionally, such discharges cause arousal as their only clinical manifestation.

Focal epileptiform discharge – a sharp wave

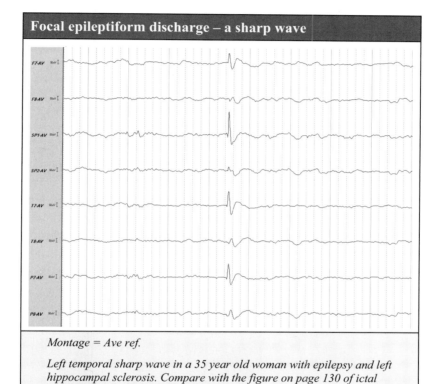

Montage = Ave ref.

Left temporal sharp wave in a 35 year old woman with epilepsy and left hippocampal sclerosis. Compare with the figure on page 130 of ictal discharge in the same patient.

Focal ictal discharge

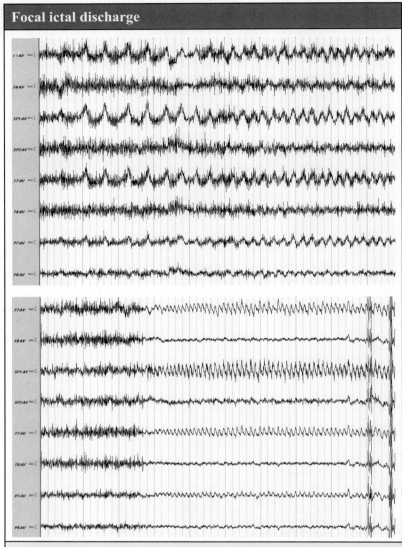

Montage = Ave ref.

Left temporal ictal discharge in the same patient on previous page.

Specific EEG Patterns in Patients with Epilepsy

Focal spikes and sharp waves

Focal epileptiform activity generally suggest focal or partial epilepsy, particularly if there is a single and consistent localization. For example, consistent right anterior temporal spikes or sharp waves suggest right anterior-mesial temporal lobe epilepsy and consistent left occipital spikes suggest left occipital lobe epilepsy.

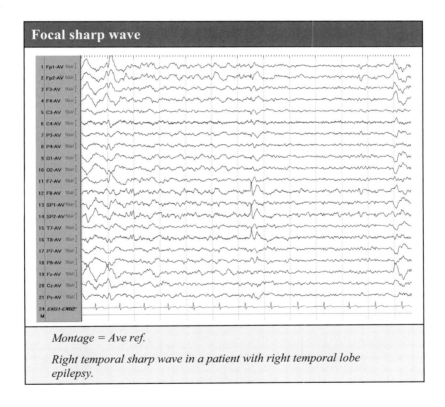

Focal sharp wave

Montage = Ave ref.

Right temporal sharp wave in a patient with right temporal lobe epilepsy.

The presence of two independent spike or sharp wave foci still suggest partial epilepsy in most instances. However, if the discharges are frontal or central they can be consistent with generalized epilepsy. In generalized epilepsy, "fragments" of generalized epileptiform discharges could be noted, particularly in sleep, in the frontal or central regions. As a rule, patients with generalized epilepsy will have generalized epileptiform discharges as well as these *fragments*.

Fragments of generalized discharges

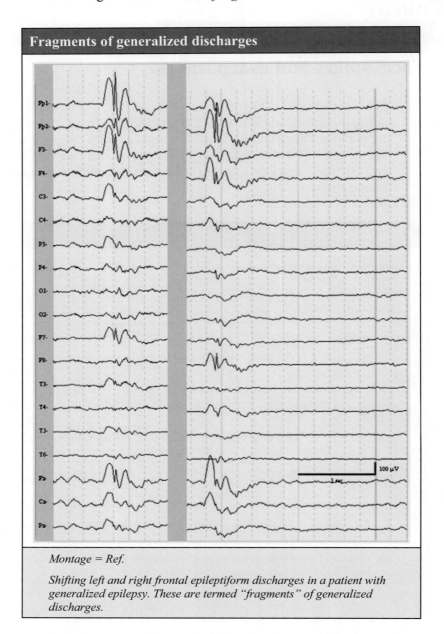

Montage = Ref.

Shifting left and right frontal epileptiform discharges in a patient with generalized epilepsy. These are termed "fragments" of generalized discharges.

Shifting asymmetries in generalized epilepsy

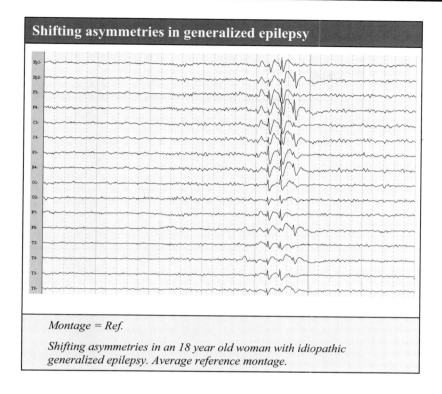

Montage = Ref.

Shifting asymmetries in an 18 year old woman with idiopathic generalized epilepsy. Average reference montage.

When there are two or more independent foci, the localization of the epileptogenic focus becomes less certain. Many patients will still have a single ictal focus, i.e. seizures may start in a single location even though interictal epileptiform activity is bilateral or even multifocal. However, patients with independent foci are more likely to have independent seizure onsets than those with single consistent foci.

Independent left and right temporal sharp waves, but single ictal focus

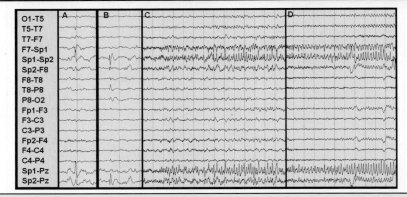

Independent left and right temporal sharp waves (A & B) but consistent left temporal seizure onsets (C&D) in a 46 year old man with intractable complex partial seizures since age 5 and left hippocampal sclerosis.

Independent left and right temporal sharp waves and independent left and right foci

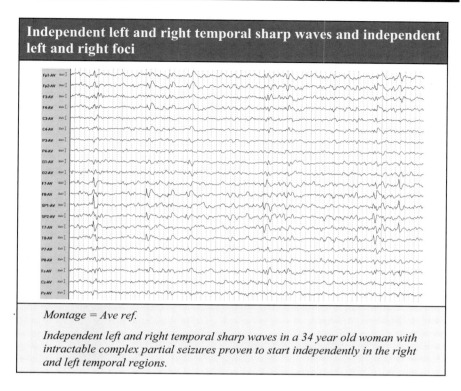

Montage = Ave ref.

Independent left and right temporal sharp waves in a 34 year old woman with intractable complex partial seizures proven to start independently in the right and left temporal regions.

3 Hz generalized spike-and-wave discharges (range 2.5 to 4 Hz)

The *3 Hz spike-and-wave discharge* suggests generalized epilepsy. If the discharges are noted in rhythmic, regular, synchronous, and symmetrical trains, they are strongly suggestive of the presence of generalized absence seizures. Specifically, they suggest typical absence seizures. Typical absence seizures generally correspond to normal intelligence and normal neurological status. As mentioned above, duration of 3 seconds or more is usually needed for seizures to be noticed by observers. Occasionally, however, the presence of motor manifestations in these seizures can make shorter discharges associated with clinically detectable seizures. In sleep, generalized spike-and-wave discharges tend to become irregular and longer in duration. In addition, there is frequent change in morphology to generalized polyspike-and-wave discharges. Therefore, the appearance of these discharges in sleep cannot predict the appearance in waking.

Generalized 3 Hz spike-and-wave activity

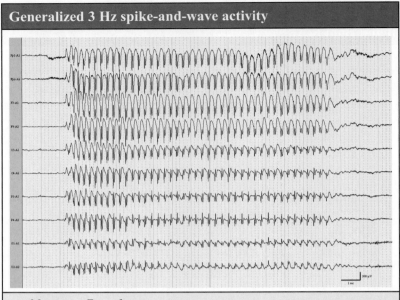

Montage = Ear ref.

Absence seizure in 9 year old girl with spells of staring and unresponsiveness for one year. She averaged 2 to 3 attacks per day, lasting seconds to 1 minute.

Regular spike-and-wave activity in waking- Irregular polyspike-and-wave discharges in sleep

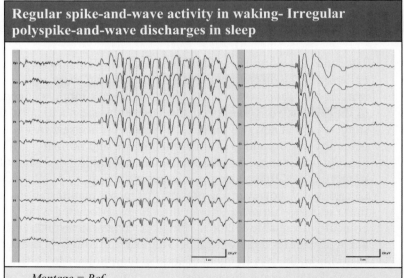

Montage = Ref

19 year old with absence seizures since age 13. Spike-and-wave discharges were regular in waking but become irregular polyspike-and-wave discharges in sleep.

Slow spike-and-wave discharges

A frequency of generalized spike-and-wave discharges below 2.5 Hz results in the term *slow spike-and-wave* or *atypical spike-and-wave*. This should be based on the frequency of discharges in waking and not in sleep. Slow spike-and-wave discharges are suggestive of symptomatic generalized epilepsy such as Lennox-Gastaut syndrome. They are associated with brain damage, and clinically correlated with atypical absence seizures. Atypical absence seizures are clinically very similar to typical absence seizures except that they may have a lesser alteration of consciousness or responsiveness with them, may have a slower onset and a more gradual termination, as well as more prominent motor features. Slow spike-and-wave discharges are more often asymmetrical and may be associated with focal epileptiform and non-epileptiform abnormalities.

Slow spike-and-wave complexes

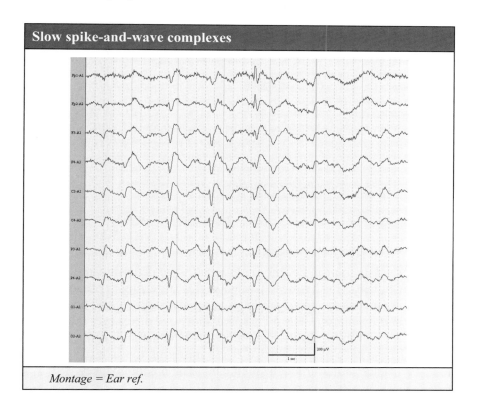

Montage = Ear ref.

Fast spike-and-wave discharges

Discharges that are faster than 4 Hz are called *fast spike-and-wave* discharges. These typically range from 4 to 7 Hz. They are seen in association with juvenile myoclonic epilepsy, but may also be seen with other generalized idiopathic epilepsies, even without myoclonic seizures. Fast spike-and-wave discharges tend to be irregular and tend to occur in clusters. These clusters can be associated with myoclonic seizures or could be subclinical/interictal. In juvenile myoclonic epilepsy, they are most likely to be recorded after arousal, particularly following sleep deprivation.

Fast spike-and-wave discharges

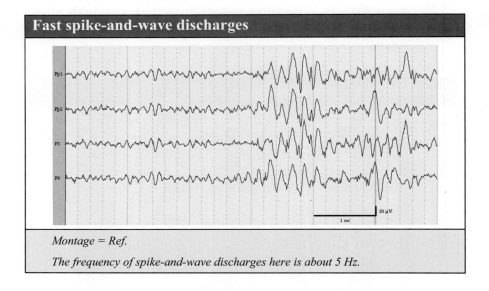

Montage = Ref.

The frequency of spike-and-wave discharges here is about 5 Hz.

The 6 Hz spike-and-wave discharges recorded in the posterior head region can be a normal variant, seen predominately in young women. This has been termed FOLD (referring to preponderance in *f*emales, *o*ccipital predominance, *l*ow-voltage, and occurrence in *d*rowsiness). The 6 Hz spike-and-wave discharges that are anterior in localization are more likely associated with epilepsy. These have been termed WHAM (referring to *w*aking, *h*igh voltage, *a*nterior localization, and *m*ale predominance).

Hypsarrhythmia

The pattern of hypsarrhythmia is commonly associated with infantile spasms, but not necessarily so. This pattern is characterized by high voltage irregular slow activity with multifocal spikes and sharp waves and periods of generalized attenuation. These periods of generalized attenuation may be without any clinical accompaniment or may be associated with infantile spasms.

Hypsarrhythmia

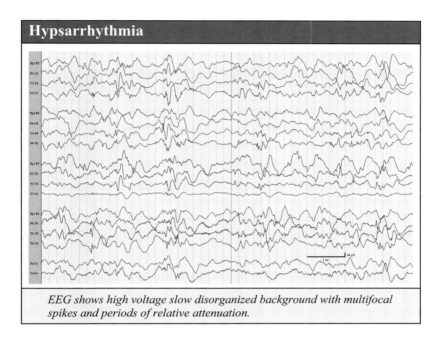

EEG shows high voltage slow disorganized background with multifocal spikes and periods of relative attenuation.

Focal ictal discharges

Ictal discharges in association with partial epilepsy typically involve rhythmic activity that evolves in frequency, morphology, voltage and distribution. Although it is most common for discharges to gradually decrease in frequency between their onset and their termination, it is not unusual for the frequency to fluctuate, increasing and then decreasing. However, towards the end of the seizure there is almost always a reduction in frequency prior to termination. The end of the seizure is sometimes clear-cut and at other times is not. The postictal slow activity can occasionally be difficult to distinguish from the rhythmic ictal activity towards the end of the seizure, which can also be in the delta range.

Focal ictal discharges may start with voltage attenuation. If this attenuation is focal, it has a localizing value. At other times, the attenuation is diffuse and less useful. The presence of high frequency beta range activity at seizure onset suggests neocortical involvement. Hippocampal seizures will typically start in the theta range, and infrequently in the alpha range. Seizure onset in the delta range may suggest that the center of seizure activity is at some distance from where the delta activity is recorded. In the case of temporal lobe epilepsy, a theta discharge in the anterior-mesial temporal region should be seen within 30 seconds of ictal onset. If not, the temporal localization is less than certain.

Focal ictal discharge

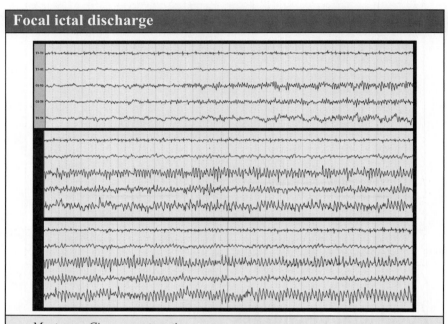

Montage = Circum, post portion.

Three consecutive 10-second EEG segments showing onset and initial evolution of a right occipital ictal discharge. The evolution included increase in voltage, decrease in frequency, and widening of the field.

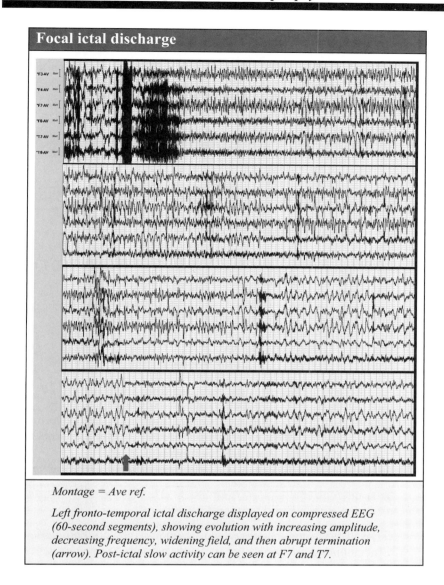

Focal ictal discharge

Montage = Ave ref.

Left fronto-temporal ictal discharge displayed on compressed EEG (60-second segments), showing evolution with increasing amplitude, decreasing frequency, widening field, and then abrupt termination (arrow). Post-ictal slow activity can be seen at F7 and T7.

TIRDA (temporal intermittent rhythmic delta activity)

This pattern is not ictal in nature. It seems to be quite specific for temporal lobe epilepsy. It is different from intermittent irregular delta activity, which is very non-specific. Although TIRDA is not yet considered epileptiform in most textbooks, the EEG interpreter may comment that this pattern is strongly associated with potential epileptogenicity.

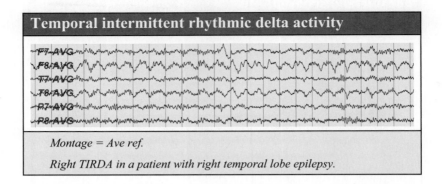

Temporal intermittent rhythmic delta activity

F7-AVG
F8-AVG
T7-AVG
T8-AVG
P7-AVG
P8-AVG

Montage = Ave ref.

Right TIRDA in a patient with right temporal lobe epilepsy.

Patterns of EEG Activity in Certain Forms of Epilepsy

Temporal lobe epilepsy

Temporal lobe epilepsy may be associated with a normal first EEG in about 50% of instances. With repeated recordings, approximately 90% of patients will demonstrate epileptiform abnormalities. There will be approximately 10% of patients who will always have a normal EEG between seizures.

Irregular delta activity may be the only EEG abnormality in some patients with temporal lobe epilepsy. This is typically recorded from the anterior-mid temporal region.

TIRDA is strongly suggestive of temporal-lobe epileptogenicity. Spikes-and-sharp waves are typically activated in drowsiness and sleep and also increase after the occurrence of seizures, particularly after the occurrence of secondarily generalized tonic-clonic seizures. As a result, in patients whose EEGs are repeatedly normal, one should try to obtain an EEG shortly after a seizure. This can help with the appearance of postictal slow activity as well as activation of epileptiform discharges. In mesial temporal lobe epilepsy, spikes-and-sharp waves will typically have prominence anteriorly at F7 or F8. If T1/T2 electrodes are used, they may have the highest field or the highest amplitude. If sphenoidal electrodes are used, they often have the highest field or the highest amplitude. There are some patients who have discharges only recorded from the sphenoidal electrodes.

Focal sharp waves and slow activity in the left sphenoidal electrode

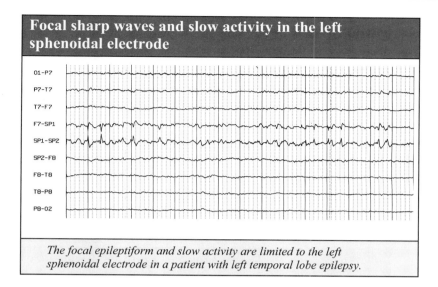

O1–P7

P7–T7

T7–F7

F7–SP1

SP1–SP2

SP2–F8

F8–T8

T8–P8

P8–O2

The focal epileptiform and slow activity are limited to the left sphenoidal electrode in a patient with left temporal lobe epilepsy.

Approximately one third of patients with temporal lobe epilepsy have independent bitemporal discharges, particularly in sleep. It is very common that during sleep the field of epileptiform discharges widens and mirror foci appear. If unilateral focal spike activity is seen in waking and an independent contralateral discharge is noted only in sleep, the waking activity is the most reliable for localization of the seizure focus. In REM sleep there is also a narrowing of the field and attenuation of mirror foci. Therefore, in patients with bilateral independent epileptiform discharges, those interictal epileptiform discharges recorded in waking or REM sleep are the most reliable for localization.

Most patients with bitemporal independent epileptiform discharges will have unilateral seizure onsets, but they have a greater chance of independent bitemporal seizure onsets than patients with unilateral epileptiform discharges. If ictal discharges are unilateral, the side with the highest frequency of epileptiform discharges is typically the side of seizure onset. A small proportion of patients may have generalized spike-and-wave discharges. This is not unexpected as a high proportion of patients may have a family history of epilepsy as well as a history of febrile convulsions early in life. The generalized spike-and-wave discharges are suspected to be an inherited EEG trait.

Simple partial seizures of temporal origin are most often not associated with EEG changes. If they are, the EEG changes tend to be subtle and quite focal.

Simple partial seizures of left temporal origin

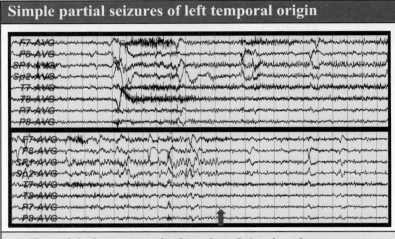

The ictal discharge is very focal, involving Sp1 and to a lesser extent Sp2. The subtle ictal discharge could have been missed without the termination.

Complex partial seizures are almost always associated with a clear-cut ictal discharge. In mesial temporal lobe epilepsy, the ictal discharge is in the theta range at onset or shortly after onset. If sphenoidal electrodes are used, an at least 5 Hz rhythmic activity noted in one sphenoidal electrode within 30 seconds of seizure onset is strongly supportive of lateralization and localization. In secondarily generalized tonic-clonic seizures of temporal lobe origin, the same EEG changes are seen early on, but the ictal discharges become generalized and the resultant muscle artifact masks the EEG.

Ictal onset in a patient with right hippocampal sclerosis

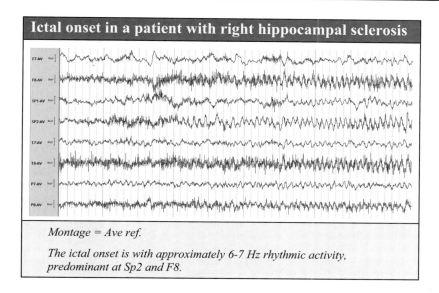

Montage = Ave ref.

The ictal onset is with approximately 6-7 Hz rhythmic activity, predominant at Sp2 and F8.

It may be difficult to distinguish neocortical from mesial temporal lobe epilepsy. If sphenoidal electrodes are used, temporal lobe ictal activity not represented in the sphenoidal electrode may favor a lateral temporal onset. Other ictal features that could suggest a neocortical temporal lobe epilepsy include a widespread hemispheric ictal onset, a delta pattern at onset without 5 Hz activity within 30 seconds of onset, and onset with periodic sharp waves. With a neocortical origin, there may be more rapid spread of the ictal discharge to extratemporal regions, and the discharge is more often bilateral at onset. A high-frequency beta range activity at onset favors a neocortical localization close to the recording electrode. However, a temporal beta-frequency discharge could represent an extratemporal origin.

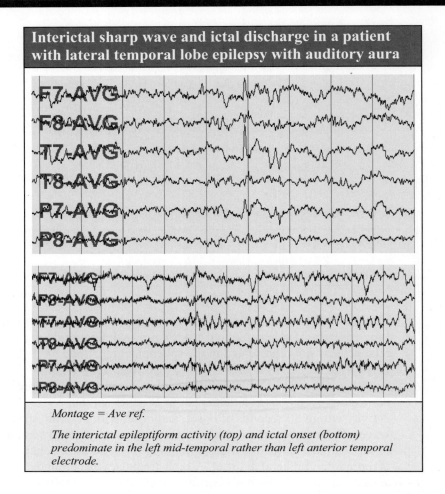

Interictal sharp wave and ictal discharge in a patient with lateral temporal lobe epilepsy with auditory aura

Montage = Ave ref.

The interictal epileptiform activity (top) and ictal onset (bottom) predominate in the left mid-temporal rather than left anterior temporal electrode.

Posterior temporal lobe epilepsy

In posterior temporal lobe epilepsy the interictal epileptiform discharges tend to have predominance in the posterior or midtemporal electrodes, and not in the anterior temporal region or the sphenoidal electrodes. The field may involve the parietal or occipital electrodes. Ictal discharge onset also tends to predominate in the posterior temporal region and not involve the sphenoidal electrodes. However, interictal epileptiform activity and ictal onset may be falsely localized. Some patients with posterior temporal lobe epilepsy may have only anterior-inferomesial temporal sharp waves, or both posterior temporal and anterior-inferomesial temporal epileptiform activity. In these patients ictal discharges may also appear to be anterior-mesial temporal. In patients with posterior temporal lesions, such false localization have historically resulted in surgical sparing of the lesion and resection of the anterior temporal and hippocampal regions, with poor surgical results.

MRI and interictal EEG in a patient with epilepsy and a left posterior temporal cavernoma

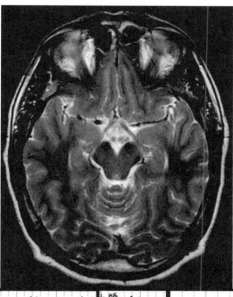

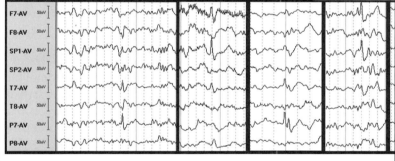

Interictal epileptiform discharges in this patient included both anterior-inferomesial temporal sharp waves (Sp1 and F7) and posterior-mid temporal spikes (P7 and T7).

Falsely localizing ictal discharge in posterior temporal lobe epilepsy

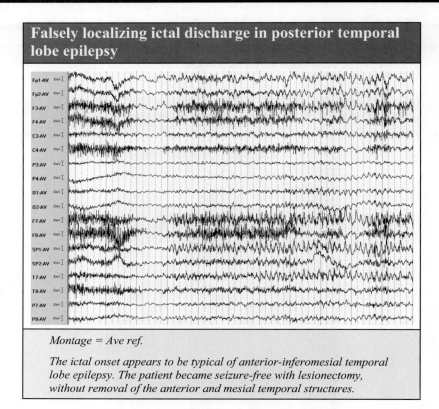

Montage = Ave ref.

The ictal onset appears to be typical of anterior-inferomesial temporal lobe epilepsy. The patient became seizure-free with lesionectomy, without removal of the anterior and mesial temporal structures.

Frontal lobe epilepsy

The frontal lobe is the largest cerebral lobe and has surfaces that are invisible or relatively invisible to EEG. Orbitofrontal onset seizures and mesial frontal onset seizures may have essentially no surface EEG manifestations. In orbitofrontal epilepsy epileptiform discharges may be recorded from the frontopolar electrodes or from supraorbital electrodes. In mesial frontal lobe epilepsy, the midline electrodes or parasagittal electrodes may record epileptiform discharges. On occasion, these discharges can be confused with vertex waves during sleep. Their occurrence in waking can help resolve this confusion. Anterior lateral frontal, dorsolateral frontal, and central foci can be associated with focal spike discharges in these regions.

Frontal lobe discharges

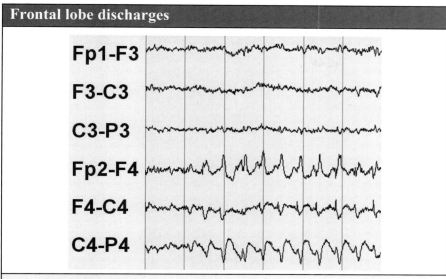

Montage = LB, subset

Right frontal spike-and-wave discharges in a patient with a right frontal convexity epileptogenic focus. There is reversal of polarity of discharges at F4.

Sharp wave predominating at the vertex in a patient with supplementary motor seizures

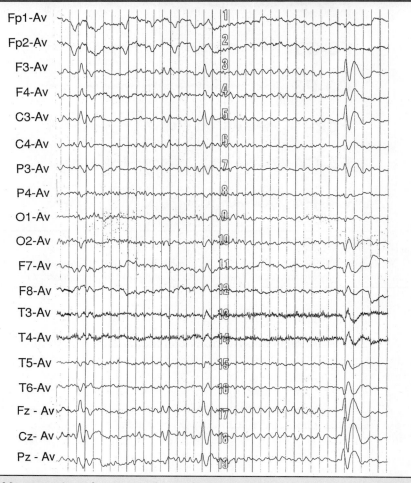

Fp1-Av		1
Fp2-Av		2
F3-Av		3
F4-Av		4
C3-Av		5
C4-Av		6
P3-Av		7
P4-Av		8
O1-Av		9
O2-Av		10
F7-Av		11
F8-Av		12
T3-Av		13
T4-Av		14
T5-Av		15
T6-Av		16
Fz - Av		17
Cz- Av		18
Pz - Av		19

Montage = Ave ref.

The sharp waves are predominant at Cz. These are not vertex waves because the patient is awake.

Supplementary motor seizure.

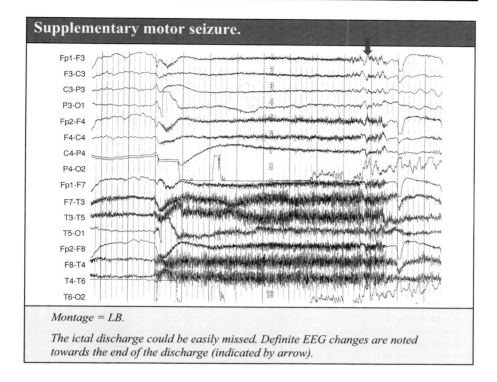

Montage = LB.

The ictal discharge could be easily missed. Definite EEG changes are noted towards the end of the discharge (indicated by arrow).

Secondary bilateral synchrony commonly occurs in frontal epilepsy. This is to be distinguished from primary bilateral synchrony seen in generalized epilepsy. Secondary bilateral synchrony can be suspected when bilateral discharges have a consistent asymmetry or a consistent lead on one side, when some focal discharges are seen only on one side, or when a consistent focal slow abnormality is seen.

Suspected secondary bilateral synchrony

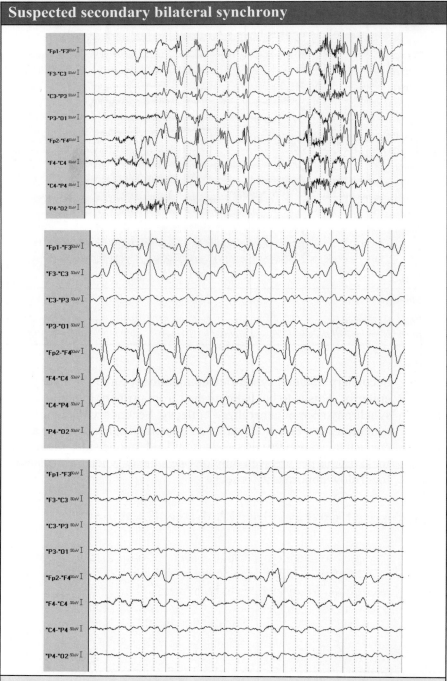

Montage = LB

There is a lead on the right in the discharge (top), a consistent asymmetry is noted with right predominance (top and middle), and right frontal slow activity is noted intermittently.

Frontal lobe seizures have a tendency to become rapidly generalized. Seizure spread is at times so fast that a focal onset could be hard to distinguish. The presence of high frequency focal fast activity at seizure onset suggests good localization of the seizure focus to the region of fast activity.

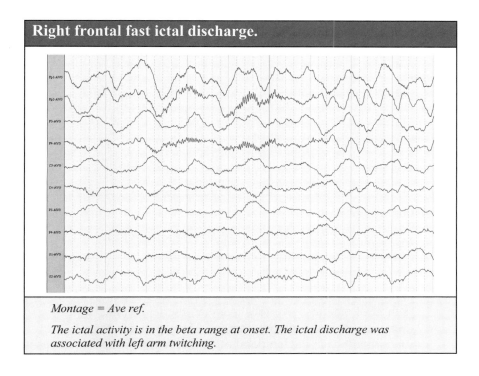

Right frontal fast ictal discharge.

Montage = Ave ref.

The ictal activity is in the beta range at onset. The ictal discharge was associated with left arm twitching.

Occipital and parietal lobe epilepsies

Occipital lobe epilepsy can be associated with focal spike or spike-and-wave discharges in the occipital region. It is not uncommon for discharges to be bilateral, since volume conduction occurs at the occipital poles (as it does at the frontal poles). Occipital lobe seizures can develop focally or regionally, or can spread to frontal or temporal lobe regions. Seizures starting above the calcarine fissure tend to spread to the frontal lobe whereas seizures starting below the calcarine fissure tend to spread to the temporal lobe. Occipital lobe seizures that remain regional have a tendency to develop very slowly, starting with beta range activity that gradually evolves to alpha range and then theta range and then delta range, over several minutes (see Figure). The progression of the ictal discharge can be so slow that the seizure may not be appreciated until the EEG has changed quite drastically.

Posterior quadrant sharp waves and ictal discharge

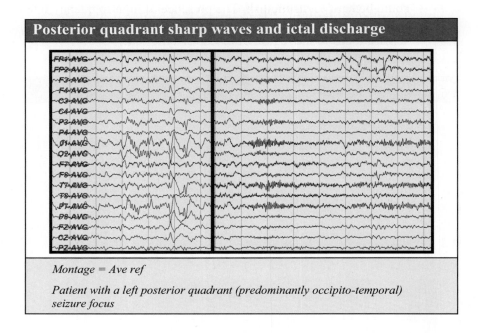

Montage = Ave ref

Patient with a left posterior quadrant (predominantly occipito-temporal) seizure focus

The EEG is often misleading in parietal lobe epilepsy. Only a subset of patients have focal parietal interictal epileptiform abnormalities and ictal discharges. Many patients have abnormalities in the temporal or frontal regions when the focus is parietal, resulting in false localization.

Benign rolandic epilepsy

In benign rolandic epilepsy, epileptiform discharges have a stereotypic appearance with broad blunt sharp waves. The classical field is negativity in the central and mid temporal regions and positivity in the bifrontal regions. However, there are common variants to this classic field. The discharges may be more posterior, involving posterior temporal and parietal regions. Some patients may have coexistent occipital lobe discharges.

Marked activation of epileptiform activity in sleep is typical. It is quite common for discharges to be recorded independently on the two sides during sleep. Awake recordings may completely miss the epileptiform activity, hence sleep is essential for diagnosis. Ictal recordings are very rare in this condition. In fact, seizures are typically a rare occurrence despite the high incidence of interictal epileptiform discharges.

Typical interictal epileptiform activity in a patient with benign rolandic epilepsy

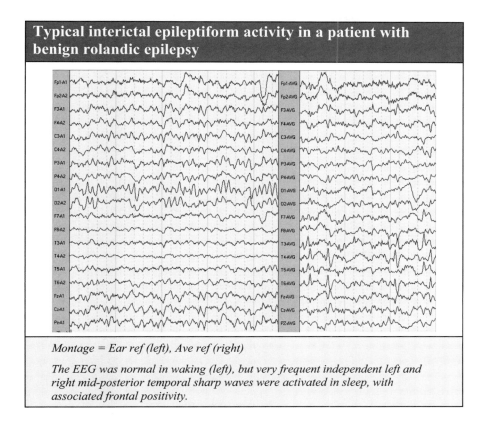

Montage = Ear ref (left), Ave ref (right)

The EEG was normal in waking (left), but very frequent independent left and right mid-posterior temporal sharp waves were activated in sleep, with associated frontal positivity.

Patients with benign rolandic epilepsy have an increased likelihood of generalized spike-and-wave discharges. Some patients may even have typical absence seizures. In such instances, it may be somewhat difficult to identify the specific clinical syndrome, as to whether it is benign rolandic epilepsy or childhood absence epilepsy.

Generalized spike-and-wave discharge in a patient with benign rolandic epilepsy

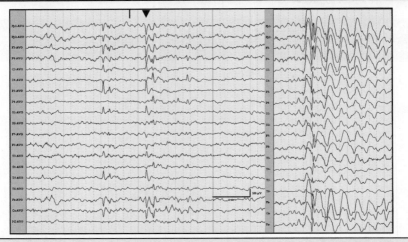

Montage = Ave ref.

The first segment to the left shows typical discharges of benign rolandic epilepsy, with bifrontal positivity (arrowhead). A generalized epileptiform discharge is seen to the right in the same patient.

Coexistent focal and generalized seizure activity

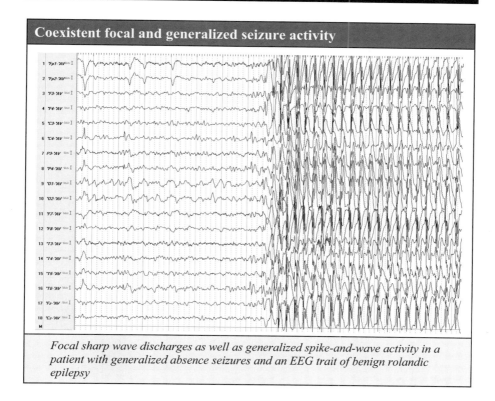

Focal sharp wave discharges as well as generalized spike-and-wave activity in a patient with generalized absence seizures and an EEG trait of benign rolandic epilepsy

Benign epilepsy with occipital paroxysms

Benign epilepsy with occipital paroxysms is characterized by high voltage spike-and-wave discharges or sharp waves recorded over the occipital and posterior temporal regions. The discharges may be unilateral or bilateral, synchronous or independent. They tend to occur in repetitive trains at times. The discharges are typically blocked by eye opening and enhanced by eye closure. They may coexist with centrotemporal or generalized spike-and-wave discharges.

Benign occipital lobe epilepsy

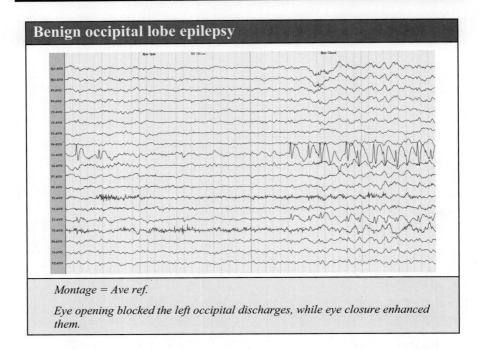

Montage = Ave ref.

Eye opening blocked the left occipital discharges, while eye closure enhanced them.

Childhood Absence Epilepsy

Childhood absence seizures are almost always precipitated by hyperventilation in untreated patients. Typical ictal discharges have a slightly faster frequency at the beginning of the seizure than at the end. They may start at 3.5-4 Hz and end at 3-2.5 Hz. The repeated spike-and-wave discharges are regular, rhythmic, synchronous and symmetrical. However, shifting asymmetries are not unusual, particularly at onset. It is not uncommon for the onset to appear one-sided for the first spike-and-wave discharge, but with sufficient number of discharges recorded, a contralateral onset will usually be seen. Postictal slow activity after the end of the generalized absence seizure is usually absent, but may occasionally be present for up to one second. The duration of generalized absence seizures is typically less than 15 seconds.

The interictal EEG background is usually normal, but OIRDA (occipital intermittent rhythmic delta activity) can be seen, at times with subtle embedded spikes or with more clear-cut bioccipital spike-and-wave activity. Fragments of generalized discharges may be seen, typically shifting between the left and right frontocentral regions.

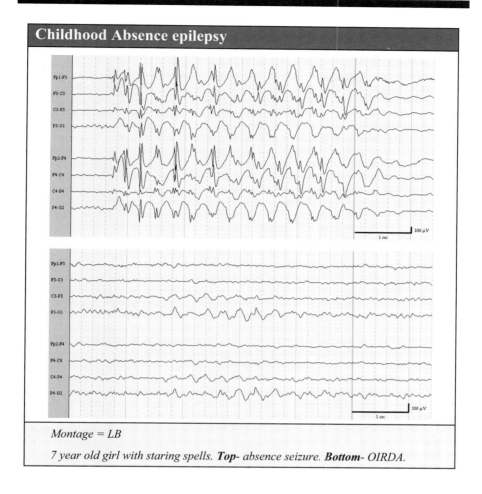

Childhood Absence epilepsy

Montage = LB

7 year old girl with staring spells. **Top-** *absence seizure.* **Bottom-** *OIRDA.*

Juvenile Absence Epilepsy

The EEG pattern of juvenile absence epilepsy is quite similar to that of childhood absence epilepsy, except that seizures are less reliably precipitated by hyperventilation and are less frequent.

Juvenile Absence Epilepsy

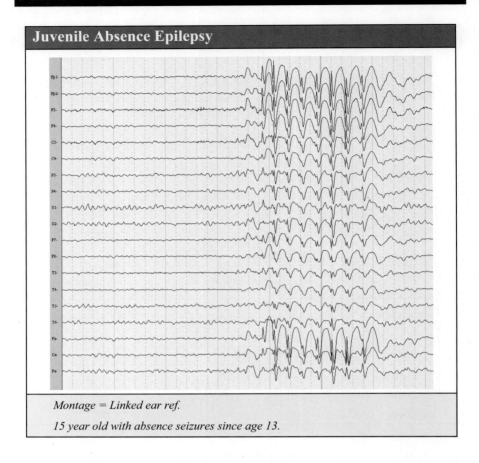

Montage = Linked ear ref.

15 year old with absence seizures since age 13.

Juvenile Myoclonic Epilepsy (JME)

In JME, fast 4–6-Hz spike-and-wave discharges and polyspike-and-wave discharges are seen interictally as well as with generalized myoclonic seizures. These discharges are more likely to occur just after arousal from sleep, especially after sleep deprivation. The background is typically normal.

About 30% of patients with JME have generalized absence seizures, and the associated EEG activity is that of typical 3-4 Hz spike-and-wave discharge.

Some focality is acceptable in this condition. Focal slow waves, spikes and sharp waves and even focal onset of the generalized discharges are present in approximately one-third of patients. In one study, in more than half the patients at least one EEG showed focal abnormalities.

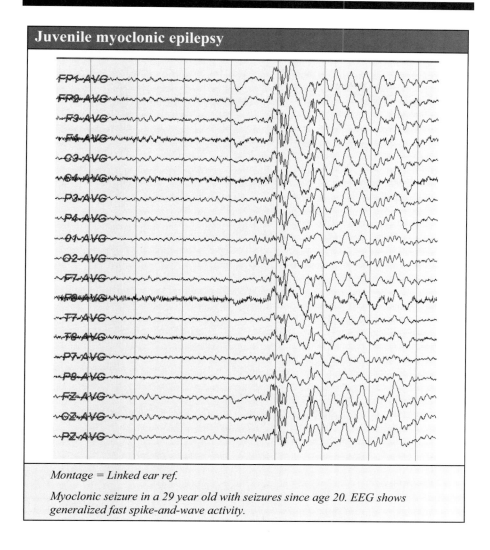

Juvenile myoclonic epilepsy

Montage = Linked ear ref.

Myoclonic seizure in a 29 year old with seizures since age 20. EEG shows generalized fast spike-and-wave activity.

Lennox-Gastaut Syndrome

Lennox-Gastaut syndrome is often characterized by a slow posterior background and with an excess of slow activity intermingled in the background. Slowing can be focal and generalized. Slow generalized spike-and-wave activity at 1.5-2 Hz is the hallmark of the condition. This may have asymmetries. In addition, there may be coexistent focal epileptiform activity. In sleep, there may be bursts of generalized polyspike activity, also called paroxysmal fast activity. These can be subclinical, or could be associated with generalized tonic seizures.

Adult Lennox-Gastaut syndrome.

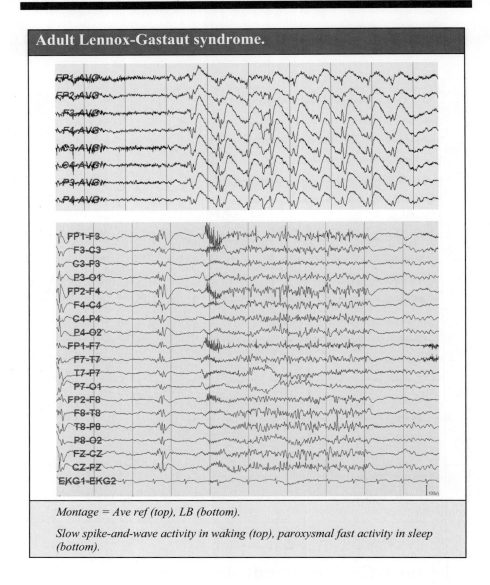

Montage = Ave ref (top), LB (bottom).

Slow spike-and-wave activity in waking (top), paroxysmal fast activity in sleep (bottom).

The EEG with Specific Seizure Types

Simple Partial Seizures

The EEG is normal in 60 to 80% of patients with simple partial seizures, even in the presence of overt motor activity, as long as the motor activity is focal and not associated with altered consciousness. In some patients, the EEG may show periodic sharp activity or very focal rhythmic activity that can be limited to only a few electrodes.

Simple partial seizure

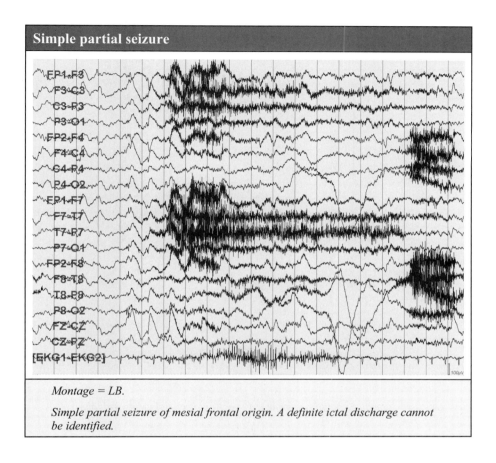

Montage = LB.

Simple partial seizure of mesial frontal origin. A definite ictal discharge cannot be identified.

Complex Partial Seizures

Complex partial seizures are almost always associated with changes on the EEG. However, if the seizures are of mesial frontal or orbitofrontal origin, they may be essentially without scalp EEG change. Artifact may mask subtle abnormal EEG activity.

On the other hand, complex partial seizures of temporal lobe origin or originating in other regions of the cerebral convexities will more often exhibit EEG changes. They tend to be more widespread than noted in simple partial seizures. In fact, they can be so widespread that a focal onset could be difficult to appreciate. This is more likely the case in extratemporal seizures, which can spread very rapidly to appear bilateral.

Complex partial seizure

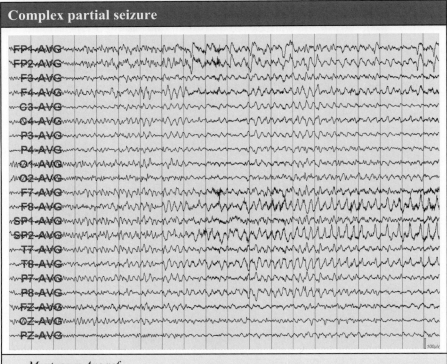

Montage = Ave ref.

Onset of a complex partial seizure in a 49 year old with right temporal lobe epilepsy.

Secondarily Generalized Tonic-Clonic Seizures

The focal onset of secondarily generalized tonic-clonic seizures determines the initial manifestations. The secondary generalization can occur early or late depending on the site of seizure origin; mesial temporal foci tend to be later.

At the time of secondary generalization muscle artifact will usually dominate the EEG. Even though the EEG is not visible, the pattern of muscle artifact can be strongly suggestive of the tonic phase and then of the clonic phase. In the clonic phase, there is typically an increased interval between muscular contractions as the seizure progresses. At the end of the muscular contractions, the EEG can show generalized attenuation or in some instances ictal activity can continue without muscular contractions.

Evolution in a secondarily generalized tonic-clonic seizure

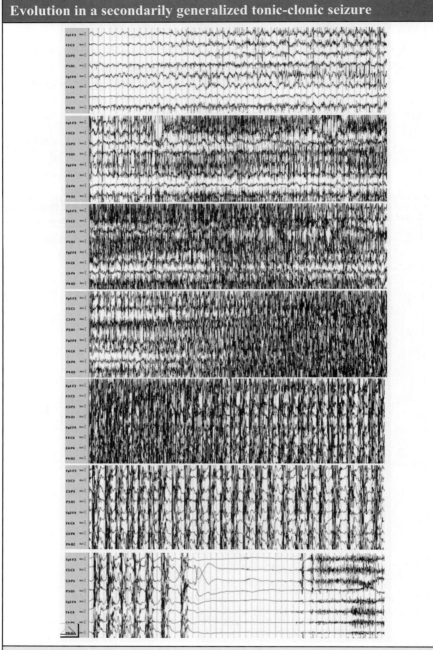

Montage = LB

Evolution in the parasagittal chains. Although the EEG is dominated by artifact, the evolution is very typical. The first arrow indicates the timing of generalized tonic phase and the second arrow the timing of the generalized clonic phase.

Generalized Absence Seizures

Generalized absence seizures were described above under the generalized childhood epilepsy syndrome. Typical generalized absence seizures will usually consist of generalized high voltage, frontally dominant, synchronous, symmetrical, regular and rhythmic 2.5-4 Hz spike-and-wave activity. There is often a faster frequency at onset, with a drop of 0.5-1 Hz towards the end of the seizure. The duration is typically less than 15 seconds and there is no postictal slowing beyond one second of termination.

Generalized absence seizure

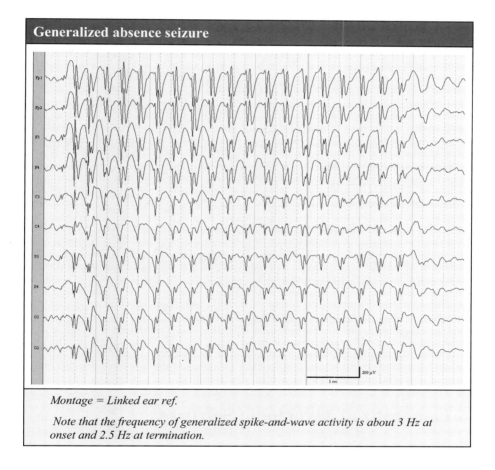

Montage = Linked ear ref.

Note that the frequency of generalized spike-and-wave activity is about 3 Hz at onset and 2.5 Hz at termination.

Generalized Atypical Absence Seizures

Generalized atypical absence seizures may have a frequency of less than 2.5 Hz. They may have slight postictal slow activity. Asymmetries are more common than with typical absence seizures. There may also be more regional distribution anteriorly. In general, the likelihood of loss of awareness decreases when the discharge becomes more regional bifrontally or bifrontocentrally.

Atypical absence seizure

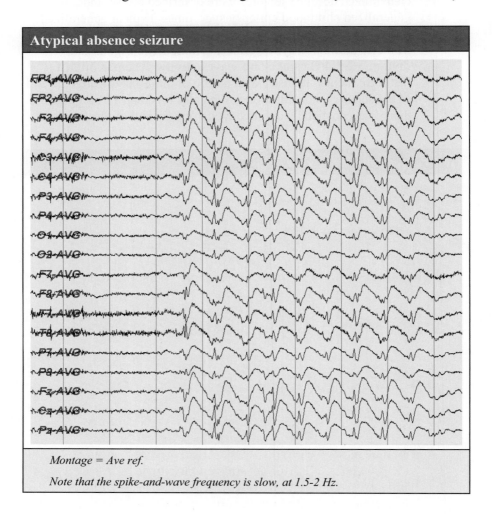

Montage = Ave ref.

Note that the spike-and-wave frequency is slow, at 1.5-2 Hz.

Generalized Myoclonic Seizures

Generalized myoclonic seizures are associated with single or a brief bursts of generalized spike-and-wave or polyspike-and-wave activity.

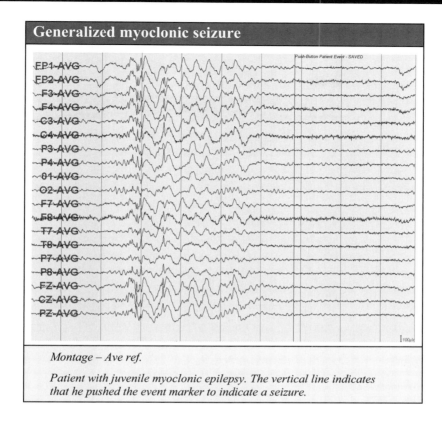

Generalized myoclonic seizure

Montage – Ave ref.

Patient with juvenile myoclonic epilepsy. The vertical line indicates that he pushed the event marker to indicate a seizure.

Generalized Tonic Seizures

Generalized tonic seizures vary in EEG manifestations. There may only be generalized attenuation. At times, the EEG is dominated with muscle artifact. There may be a generalized 10 Hz rhythmic activity or generalized high-frequency low-voltage activity. Tonic seizures are generally short. Slow activity may become intermixed progressively during the seizure progression. There may be postictal slow activity.

Generalized tonic seizure

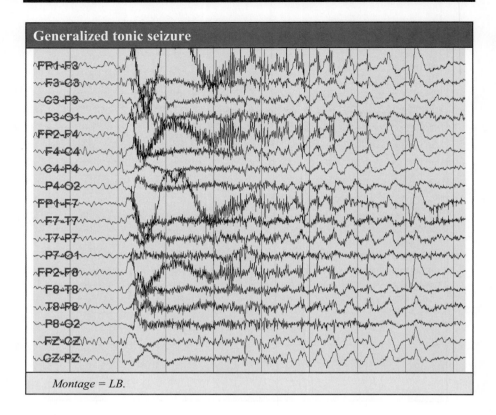

Montage = LB.

Generalized Atonic Seizures

Generalized atonic seizures can have a similar EEG appearance to generalized tonic seizures, when they occur in patients with Lennox-Gastaut syndrome or other symptomatic generalized epileptic syndromes. If they occur in the setting of myoclonic astatic epilepsy, they tend to include a generalized spike-and-wave discharge or burst followed by a large slow wave with generalized attenuation of faster activity for 1 to 3 seconds.

Generalized atonic seizure in a patient with Lennox-Gastaut

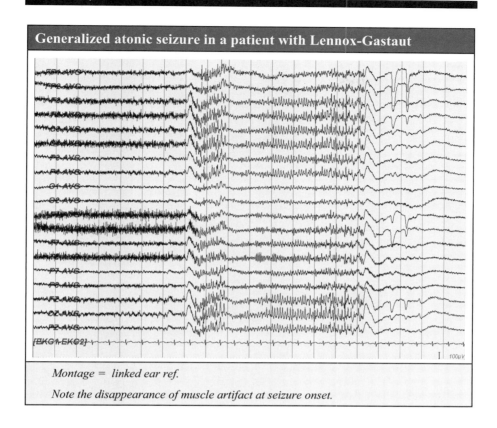

Montage = linked ear ref.

Note the disappearance of muscle artifact at seizure onset.

Generalized myoclonic-atonic seizure

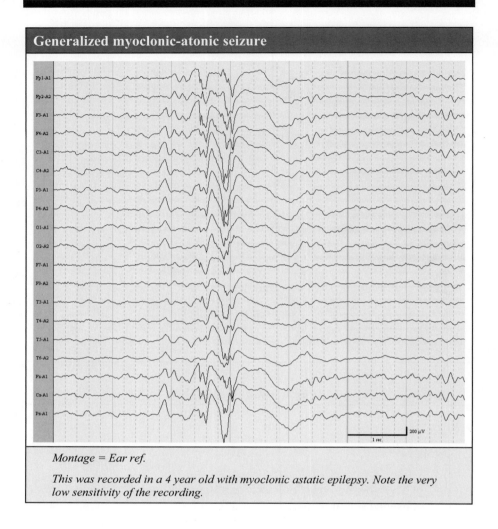

Montage = Ear ref.

This was recorded in a 4 year old with myoclonic astatic epilepsy. Note the very low sensitivity of the recording.

Infantile Spasm

Infantile spasms are associated with generalized attenuation, which may have superimposed beta or alpha range activity. These are typically quite brief, lasting sometimes less than one second. The interictal EEG is usually high voltage, so that the attenuation is easy to note.

Infantile spasm

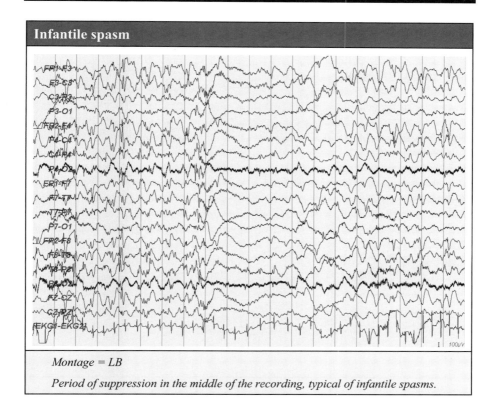

Montage = LB

Period of suppression in the middle of the recording, typical of infantile spasms.

Generalized Tonic-Clonic Seizures .

Generalized tonic-clonic seizures may evolve from generalized absence seizures or generalized myoclonic seizures, or they may start as generalized tonic-clonic seizures. If they evolve from a previous different seizure type, there is typically evolution to high-frequency rhythmic activity. Generally, the EEG becomes dominated by muscle artifact. However, in the absence of muscle artifact or underneath muscle artifact, there is usually evolution to approximately 10 Hz rhythmic discharge that evolves into generalized polyspike and then polyspike-and-wave discharges that slow down in frequency before the end of the discharge. After the discharge, there is generalized voltage attenuation.

Generalized tonic-clonic seizure onset

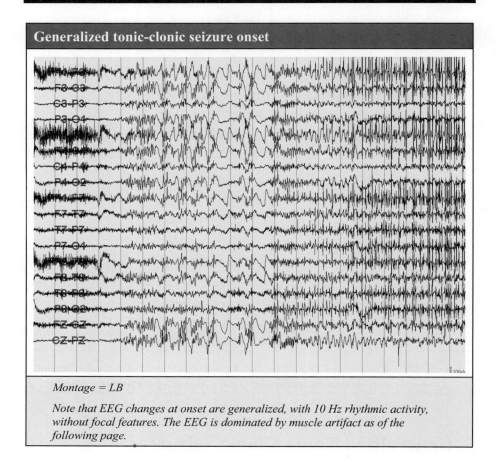

Montage = LB

Note that EEG changes at onset are generalized, with 10 Hz rhythmic activity, without focal features. The EEG is dominated by muscle artifact as of the following page.

Limitation of Routine EEG in Epilepsy

The routine EEG is an indirect assessment, seizures being an intermittent phenomenon. It relies on ictal discharges but approximately 50% of patients with epilepsy will have a normal first EEG and 10% will always have a normal interictal EEG. The interictal EEG abnormalities may be unreliable for diagnosis and classification because some patients with nonepileptic seizures may have interictal epileptiform discharges as an EEG trait. Occasionally, patients with focal epilepsy have generalized discharges, or patients with generalized epilepsy may have focal discharges, which could be misleading.

The EEG Predictive Value

Prediction of recurrence after first seizure

In patients with a single unprovoked seizure, there is a higher risk of recurrence if the EEG shows epileptiform abnormalities. Generalized spike-and-wave discharges seem to be more predictive. In a large meta-analysis, there was a twofold increase in relative risk of seizure recurrence in patients with epileptiform abnormalities in comparison with those that have a normal EEG. In a recent study, EEGs performed within 48 hours of the first seizure were even more predictive, with a 4.5 fold increase in risk of recurrence when epileptiform discharges were recorded.

Prediction of seizure recurrence after medication withdrawal

Most studies report an increased risk of relapse in patients whose EEG pattern is abnormal just before discontinuing antiepileptic drugs. However, the diagnosis of the epileptic syndrome may be a better predictor of relapse.

Specificity of the EEG

Epileptiform discharges are fairly rare in the normal nonepileptic population. The incidence has been estimated at about 0.4%. One study in nonepileptic neurologic patients revealed an incidence of 1.7%, but some of these patients went on to have seizures later on. Certain localizations of sharp waves in children have lesser significance. This includes central, mid-temporal and occipital interictal epileptiform discharges. Needle-like spikes in the occipital lobe may occur in children with congenital blindness and have weak association with epilepsy (epilepsy occurs in approximately one-half of patients with occipital spikes but one-third of those with early onset visual deprivation). Relatives of patients with benign rolandic epilepsy may have centrotemporal spikes in the absence of any epilepsy. In newborns, particularly in premature newborns, multifocal spikes may be normal and have no association with epilepsy. Generalized spike-and-wave discharges may occur in asymptomatic siblings of children with generalized absence seizures and may be inherited as an EEG trait. A photoparoxysmal response is often seen in the absence of epilepsy. For example, photosensitivity was found in 0.72% of newly recruited entrants for training as pilots.

In practice, the most common reason for false positive EEGs is misinterpretation of normal EEG findings, particularly in drowsiness, and less often misinterpretation of incidental or irrelevant EEG abnormalities. The sources of erroneous epileptiform interpretation include artifacts, normal sharp activity in drowsiness, in particular wicket spikes, third rhythm, Mu rhythm and fragments of the Mu rhythm. Another source of potential misinterpretation is that of benign variants discussed earlier (see Chapter 5).

Chapter 8.
Video EEG

Video EEG is divided into short-duration and long-duration studies. Short-duration studies are performed usually on outpatients although inpatients can also be studied. Short-duration studies are used predominantly to differentiate seizures from pseudoseizures.

Prolonged Video-EEG Monitoring

Clinical indications for video-EEG

Prolonged video-EEG monitoring was developed for more direct evaluation of seizures. The 20-minute "routine" EEG is only an indirect assessment in patients with seizures and spells of unknown nature. Aside from select syndromes such as childhood absence epilepsy and benign epilepsy with centrotemporal spikes, the interictal EEG is often normal in patients with epilepsy. Studies estimate that approximately 50% of patients with epilepsy may have a normal initial EEG. Repeated EEG studies increase that number to about 90%. Therefore, a proportion of patients will always have a normal interictal EEG.

If the diagnosis of epilepsy was assured clinically, treatment could proceed without the need for EEG evidence. However, when seizures do not respond to initial therapy, doubts arise regarding the certainty of the epilepsy diagnosis or the certainty of epilepsy classification. The most solid clinical diagnosis requires the ability to witness and analyze a typical seizure and its EEG correlate. The technology of video-EEG allows capturing of events and provides ability to replay seizures for detailed analysis of the clinical signs and the corresponding EEG changes.

The main indications for video-EEG monitoring are:

- *Diagnosis of atypical seizures or spells of unknown nature.* The need for video EEG could arise because events are atypical for seizures, because there has been absence of evidence for epilepsy by history and by tests, because there has been no response to antiepileptic drug (AED) therapy, or because a patient with known epilepsy started having new "different" spells.
- *Accurate classification of seizures for optimal choice of medical therapy.* This situation applies to individuals with documented epilepsy in whom there may be incomplete or contradictory clinical and EEG data for classification purposes. An example of this would include an adolescent with staring spells and an EEG that shows both focal and generalized discharges. The seizures could represent generalized absence seizures, in which case the most appropriate therapy could be ethosuximide, or complex partial seizures, in which case ethosuximide would be ineffective and a medication more appropriate for partial seizures would be used.
- *Localization of the epileptogenic focus for possible surgical resection.* There is evidence to suggest that after failure of two antiepileptic drugs the chances of seizure freedom with another agent decreases. Patients who are refractory to medical therapy should be investigated for the presence of a surgically remediable epileptic syndrome.

Additional indications for video-EEG monitoring include:

- *Quantification of seizures.* Although this tends to be a research application, it could be clinically useful in counting frequent seizures, for example generalized absence seizures.
- *Quantification of response to treatment.* This is also frequently a research application, but has clinical application for checking efficacy of therapy of absence seizures in childhood absence epilepsy. In this syndrome, seizures are frequent, and the response can be quantified with a 24-hour monitoring study.
- Studying seizure precipitants described in the history.
- *Reflex epilepsy*: video-EEG monitoring can easily record seizures if the reflex precipitant can be reproduced.
- *Self-induction:* some patients have resistant seizures because of auto-induction. Video-EEG monitoring can document the occurrence of auto-induction in this situation.
- *Situational factors:* when situational factors are reported to precipitate seizures, they may potentially be reproduced in the setting of the epilepsy monitoring unit.
- Documentation of ictal and interictal discharges during circadian rhythms. This is frequently a research application.

- *Clinical correlate of EEG discharge.* Some patients have EEG discharges that could be ictal in nature. The presence or absence of clinical changes may be necessary for counseling regarding driving or other restrictions. Simultaneous video with the EEG allows testing and demonstration of changes in responsiveness or cognitive functions in conjunction with the EEG discharge.
- *Transitory cognitive impairment.* This is predominantly a research application. Very sensitive testing has allowed the demonstration of subtle dysfunction in association with interictal epileptiform discharges.
- *Finding interictal evidence for epilepsy.* This application does not necessarily require the video component.

Video-EEG monitoring choices

Possible choices for video-EEG monitoring include:

- Inpatient long-term video-EEG monitoring
- Inpatient short-term video-EEG monitoring
- Ambulatory EEG monitoring

Inpatient long-term video-EEG monitoring

This is performed in a fixed epilepsy monitoring unit. In this setting the most up-to-date equipment uses cameras fixed in the patient rooms. There is a possibility of using two cameras at different angles in different zoom settings. The electrodes attached to the patient's head are connected to a head box. Signals are amplified and transmitted through a cable to a computer that records the digitized EEG signal. The video signal is similarly digitized and synchronized.

Most epilepsy monitoring units currently use seizure and spike detection paradigms. These are extremely helpful to identify seizures that patients are not aware of, but they have a very high false-positive detection rate so that every detection has to be reviewed to determine its validity.

Patients are typically admitted for several days. If they have been on anti-epileptic drugs then these drugs are reduced or discontinued in order to facilitate the recording of seizures. Some medications have to be withdrawn carefully as they can be associated with particularly severe withdrawal seizures. This in particular has been demonstrated for carbamazepine.

Identification of seizures can be performed in several ways:

- An event marker button that the patient or patient family can push in the event of a seizure.
- Automatic seizure detection program.
- Seizure log/diary kept by the patient/family/caretaker.
- Screening the EEG or video. The latter technique can be excessively time consuming.
- Density spectral array, offered by some manufacturers. This gives a display that could identify periods in which changes are suspicious and warrant review for possible seizures. This can markedly facilitate review of EEG for possible seizures.

DSA

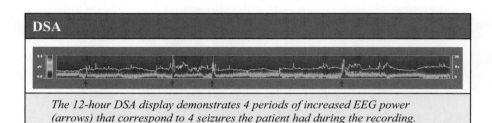

The 12-hour DSA display demonstrates 4 periods of increased EEG power (arrows) that correspond to 4 seizures the patient had during the recording.

Using a combination of all of the above, long-term video-EEG monitoring in the epilepsy monitoring unit (EMU) is successful in the vast majority of patients in recording epileptic seizures for analysis.

Repeated admissions

Occasionally, admission has to be repeated. If a second admission fails to record seizures, the approach to video-EEG monitoring may have to be modified. One of the factors that contribute to the failure of video-EEG monitoring is the elimination of daily life stressors when the patients are admitted. These stressors may be necessary to precipitate seizures. For patients with true epilepsy, withdrawal of medications may be an effective counterbalance. Some patients have cyclical seizure patterns and the video-EEG monitoring session would have the highest yield if scheduled at the next expected cycle. This is most commonly encountered in women with catamenial epilepsy in whom seizures are most likely just before or during the menstrual period. In other women, seizures are also more likely around the time of ovulation. Even men may have cyclical seizure precipitation, and the video-EEG monitoring could have a higher yield taking these into consideration.

Goals of monitoring

Monitoring for presurgical localization

If video-EEG monitoring is scheduled for the purpose of pre-surgical seizure localization, then recording of three to six seizures is usually required. In the presence of conflicting data, a larger number of seizures may be needed to resolve the conflict and to increase certainty.

Some patients have independent left and right temporal seizure onsets and these patients may still be candidates for surgery if more than 80% of seizures arise in one focus, or if only clinically insignificant seizures arise on one side and all clinically significant seizures arise on the other. In these more complicated cases a larger number of seizures may be needed for accurate classification.

In some patients with independent interictal epileptiform discharges arising on both sides, a particular cluster of seizures may come from one of the two foci. In these patients, seizures cannot be recorded solely from a single cluster. Repeat monitoring at a different point in time may be advisable to record a separate cluster of seizures.

Monitoring for differentiation of epileptic from non-epileptic spells

If the purpose of monitoring is to determine whether a seizure is epileptic or non-epileptic, the recording of a highly typical non-epileptic seizure could be sufficient for the purposes of monitoring. However, there are potential pitfalls and one should be extremely careful in the analysis of data. For many patients, recording additional seizures is advisable and continuing to record until anti-epileptic drugs have been cleared would provide further assurance. Some patients may have had epilepsy and new spells may be non-epileptic. The recording of a characteristic new spell that is non-epileptic does not necessarily eliminate the possibility of persistent controlled epilepsy.

Non-epileptic seizures are often provoked early with suggestion, whereas epileptic seizures will often appear at a latency, as anti-epileptic drugs are cleared. Some patients may erroneously identify an event as a typical seizure because they do not know what happens during a typical event. Not only can some patients with epilepsy be suggested to have a non-epileptic event, but others may spontaneously have an atypical psychogenic event in the charged suggestive environment. It is mandatory for a patient's family member to identify an event as typical. If typical events are recorded and are deemed psychogenic and nothing different happens after anti-epileptic drugs have been essentially completely cleared, then the possibility of pure psychogenic seizures is most likely. One can be most secure in this diagnosis when the onset of episodes is recent and it can be clearly confirmed that no events other than typical recorded ones have occurred in the past.

Monitoring for classification of seizure type

If the purpose of the video-EEG monitoring is to classify the seizure type, then recording of a single seizure may be sufficient if that recorded seizure has a clear focal onset and seizure semiology that agrees with the EEG localization. In other instances, however, one cannot be so certain with a single recorded seizure. In some patients, the seizure onset may appear generalized but the clinical seizure pattern may suggest a focal origin. In these instances, it may become necessary to record more than one event, in addition to interictal epileptiform activity.

Baseline EEG recording

Ideally, every session of video-EEG monitoring should be preceded by a baseline EEG. This baseline EEG provides the opportunity to record clean activity while the patient is relaxed and inactive. The posterior background rhythm can be recorded and its reactivity tested to eye opening and closure. Hyperventilation and photic stimulation should be a component of that baseline EEG.

Provocation of events

Provocation of non-epileptic seizures

The use of other suggestion techniques has been controversial. In particular, the element of deception that could be involved has been deemed unethical by some. The authors feel that suggestion does not necessarily need to involve deception. One suggestion technique that our laboratory has adopted is the use of an alcohol swab over the neck, typically in conjunction with hyperventilation. The technologist makes a statement to the patient that this can trigger seizures in some patients. This statement in itself does not involve deception. The suggestion certainly can trigger seizures in some patients, which in the vast majority are non-epileptic in origin. The use of suggestion early in the course of the study facilitates the recording of psychogenic seizures and improves the efficiency of the study.

Caution should be exercised because some patients with epilepsy are suggestible and may be driven to have events that they don't normally have. Even patients with non-epileptic seizures may have typical attacks with suggestion. Hence, the verification with family members that recorded attacks are typical of historical ones is essential. During the video-EEG monitoring study, other precipitation methods could be used. It is important to obtain a detailed history from a patient regarding any precipitating events that can be reproduced in the epilepsy monitoring unit.

Intravenous saline injection has been advocated as a suggestion method for precipitation of psychogenic seizures. This has been the main focus of the controversy regarding use of deception. The authors have a similar perspective on this technique as with other modes of suggestion. The use of saline injection is totally reasonable if the element of deception is removed. Since this requires IV access, it is generally not used during the baseline section of the recording and has been left as a method of last resort. The authors have avoided any deception by describing the injection to the patient as a saline injection and indicating that this may precipitate seizures in some patients. This method has been applied when the study is about to be concluded and no events have been recorded, while the historical evidence strongly favors a non-epileptic psychogenic basis for the attacks. The atmosphere is maximized for suggestibility with relative silence, darkness and eye closure. If there is a relative or friend available, that person is used to maximize the atmosphere of suggestibility. The patient is asked to hyperventilate and the injection is started approximately one minute later and announced by the examiner. If a tremor or other movement is noted, the examiner can communicate with the relative or friend, asking if this is a sign of a seizure starting. If the relative answers positively, that seems to facilitate the development of a full-fledged attack.

Precipitation of epileptic seizures

Withdrawal of anti-epileptic drugs is the main method of precipitation of epileptic seizures used in the monitoring unit. However, other techniques can be added on, particularly sleep deprivation. This is most effective for generalized epilepsy, particularly juvenile myoclonic epilepsy. In that condition seizures sometimes occur only in the setting of sleep deprivation and usually after arousal from premature awakening. In partial epilepsy, sleep deprivation may be less effective. In patients whose seizures are predominately in sleep, particularly patients with frontal lobe epilepsy, sleep deprivation is useful only in as far as making seizures more likely with the next session of sleep. It is best in these instances to alternate sleep deprivation and a full night's sleep. Using sleep deprivation on consecutive nights and days may not be justified or fruitful. If an ictal SPECT is planned during the session of video-EEG monitoring, sleep deprivation at night can be followed by allowing the patient to sleep during the daytime when the ictal SPECT injection is possible. This is most useful for patients whose seizures typically occur in sleep.

End of the study

When should the study end?

The video-EEG monitoring study ends once a sufficient number of seizures have been recorded and the patient has been stabilized. In patients who develop a cluster of seizures or who have generalized tonic-clonic seizures during the monitoring session, one day without seizures would be advisable before discharge. Certainly, the safety of discharge also depends on many individual factors such as whether the patient lives alone and how far the patient lives from the medical center or from an emergency department. A patient who lives alone requires a greater evidence of stability prior to discharge.

Medications upon discharge

The admission to the epilepsy monitoring unit presents an opportunity to make medication changes for many patients. For patients with documented epilepsy, the admission could be an opportunity to withdraw a medication, such as carbamazepine, that would be difficult to withdraw on outpatient basis. The inpatient setting allows a faster withdrawal and treatment of withdrawal seizures with intravenous or oral medications on an as-needed basis. For patients with non-epileptic psychogenic seizures and no evidence of epilepsy, it is most appropriate to discontinue anti-epileptic drugs prior to discharge. As a component of the treatment of patients with pure psychogenic seizures, withdrawal of anti-epileptic drugs helps remove the ambiguity about the diagnosis so that effective treatment can be pursued with psychotherapy or psychiatric medications as needed.

Short-term video-EEG monitoring

This form of video-EEG monitoring is performed for two to eight hours on either outpatient or inpatient basis. This form of monitoring avoids the need for hospital admission. It is the preferred form of monitoring for children and adults who have very frequent attacks or for patients in whom attacks can be reliably precipitated. For example, a variety of reflex epilepsies can be diagnosed on outpatient video-EEG. Examples could include photosensitive epilepsy, startle epilepsy, reading epilepsy, eating epilepsy, and musicogenic epilepsy.

If the short-term video monitoring session fails to record an attack despite the use of appropriate activation techniques, then prolonged inpatient monitoring could be performed. It is often impractical and inappropriate to make medication changes in short-term video-EEG monitoring sessions. An exception could be the individual who reports that missing a single dose of medication reliably brings on attacks, or the individual who has only very mild events that would not present a medical risk.

Ambulatory video-EEG monitoring

Ambulatory video-EEG has the advantage of keeping the patient in an environment that includes the usual stressors. Most commonly, this technology is applied without the video component. However, some manufacturers provide video in conjunction with ambulatory EEG. Concomitant video use is possible when the patient is stationary, for example working at a desk, sitting on a sofa, or sleeping.

In the absence of concomitant video, interpretation of ambulatory EEG presents many challenges. It is well known that artifact can imitate any EEG abnormality and without knowing the concomitant behavior one cannot exclude the possibility that movement or other patterns of muscle activity and behavior could be responsible. Ambulatory EEG alone would be most helpful in major attacks that involve loss of consciousness or complete loss of awareness. In these instances, the persistence of a normal EEG strongly suggests a non-epileptic, even non-organic origin of attacks. Ambulatory EEG becomes less appropriate for subtle events, in particular events that do not involve alteration of awareness. It has been established that 60 to 80% of simple partial seizures do not have an EEG correlate.

Features of different methods of monitoring			
Test	STM	LTM	Ambulatory EEG without video
Setting	Outpatient or Inpatient	Outpatient	Natural environment
Advantages	Does not require admission	Thorough	Maximal mobility, natural stressors
Key Indications	Children/ infants Frequent attacks Attacks can be precipitated	Presurgical evaluation Infrequent attacks Medication changes needed	Spells involving total loss of consciousness Attack frequency once a day Attacks requiring natural stressors
Clinical correlation	Excellent	Excellent	Inadequate

Special electrodes

Clearly diagnostic video-EEG studies may not need special electrode use. However, additional electrodes besides the 10-20 system may be very useful for localization purposes.

10-10 system

Electrodes can be added from the 10-10 system as needed depending on the specific suspected localization.

Nasopharyngeal electrodes

To record from the mesial-basal temporal cortex, nasopharyngeal electrodes were used in the past, but much less now. These electrodes can be irritating and increasingly so with the passage of time. In addition, they are unstable and likely to be dislodged with movement and when a seizure occurs. They are certainly not appropriate for long-term monitoring beyond a few hours.

Sphenoidal electrodes

Sphenoidal electrodes are extremely valuable. They have an advantage of being stable. Even though they are painful at insertion and can be associated with residual pain for the first day after insertion, they are better tolerated with the passage of time. There has been some controversy regarding their ability to provide unique information. In the opinion of the authors, there is a fraction of patients with temporal lobe epilepsy whose interictal discharges may not be visible without sphenoidal electrodes and whose ictal onsets would be a lot less well localized without them as well. In some patients, the ictal onset appears a lot more widespread until sphenoidal electrodes are used, identifying an impressive focal predominance or even a focal onset. The authors usually use sphenoidal electrodes in patients undergoing presurgical evaluation, in whom a temporal lobe origin is likely.

Alternatives to the deep sphenoidal electrodes include:

- *Mini-sphenoidal electrodes* that are inserted only 1 cm
- Zygomatic electrodes
- Cheek electrodes
- Anterior temporal (T1/T2) electrodes
- Electrode placements based on the 10-10 system that supplement the 10-20 temporal electrodes

Strictly speaking, the sphenoidal electrodes record from the mesial basal temporal region or the inferomesial temporal region, whereas zygomatic and other lateral electrodes may record from the lateral basal or inferolateral temporal region.

Supraorbital electrodes

For patients with suspected orbitofrontal seizure origin, supraorbital electrodes may enhance the recording of epileptiform activity and ictal onsets from the anterior orbitofrontal cortex.

It should be noted, however, that supraorbital electrodes will frequently record anterior temporal discharges if the dipole is oriented in an anterior-posterior direction. Therefore, the interpretation of activity originating in the supraorbital electrodes will depend on the field of this activity.

Nasoethmoidal electrodes

Nasoethmoidal electrodes for recording orbitofrontal activity are impractical as they require placement by an ENT specialist. They are seldom used in routine practice.

Review of Video-EEG studies

In reviewing video-EEG studies, the interpreter places the greatest emphasis on ictal clinical events. There are clinical and EEG features to each of these events.

Clinical features to be assessed are:

- Time of occurrence
- Activity the patient was engaged in
- Apparent precipitation
- Time of first clinical change and the nature of the first clinical change
- Evolution of clinical activity and a description of activity at each phase and its evolution
- Apparent end of the clinical event
- Duration of the clinical seizure
- The nature of postictal behavior, including interaction with examiners
- Time of return to normal functioning, if possible to determine

EEG features to be assessed are:

- State of the patient at the time the event started (e.g. waking vs sleep)
- First change in the EEG, including attenuation or disappearance of previous interictal epileptiform activity, and attenuation of previous background activity. If the attenuation is focal, this can be a useful localizing finding
- First definite rhythmic activity and its localization, its evolution and pattern of spread
- Time of complete termination of the ictal discharge. It may also be worthwhile noting when ictal activity ends in one hemisphere or in most electrodes except one region
- Postictal EEG pattern (e.g. generalized attenuation or lateralized or focal attenuation, or lateralized or focal irregular slow activity)

Filtering

The reviewer must look at the EEG unfiltered. Reviewing the ictal EEG in a filtered state first could result in misinterpretation of muscle and movement artifact as cerebral in origin, because they have lost some of their characteristic hallmarks as a result of the filtering. The pattern of muscle artifact during a seizure can be greatly helpful. For example, generalized tonic and generalized clonic motor activity both produce typical myogenic patterns on the EEG. Subtle focal clonic activity in the face can be recognized on EEG even when not obvious on video review, and chewing and swallowing artifacts can also be recognized on the EEG.

Montages

For purposes of localization and classification, seizures may need to be viewed in more than one montage. Using an initial bipolar montage, one can estimate the center of the field based on reversal of polarity. The seizure can then be viewed in a referential montage, choosing a reference that is least likely to be involved in the seizure activity. For example, the ipsilateral ear is an inappropriate reference for a seizure originating in the anterior-inferomesial temporal region, because the ear ipsilateral to the seizure origin is frequently involved in the ictal discharge. The average reference can be appropriate but may need to be manipulated to exclude the most clearly involved electrodes.

Anterior-inferomesial temporal ictal discharges rarely predominate in the midline parietal electrode (Pz), and that becomes a suitable reference. The midline has the least muscle density and therefore is likely to have the least muscle artifact. If appropriate, midline electrodes could serve as a suitable reference. Seizures that appear generalized or parasagittal can be reviewed with the ear reference with preserved fidelity. The reviewer should realize that the appearance of the seizure and its field may change remarkably with the selection of the reference. This is a clear reflection of the difficulty with finding a neutral reference. Thoughtful consideration has to be applied to select the montage that likely provides the highest fidelity.

Video-EEG diagnosis of psychogenic seizures

The simplest diagnosis of psychogenic seizures occurs in the absence of motor activity in patients who become unresponsive while still, or collapse and become unresponsive. In these patients, the presence of a completely normal EEG background while the patient is totally unresponsive would be diagnostic of a non-organic psychogenic activity.

A positive diagnosis of non-epileptic psychogenic seizures becomes harder in the presence of associated motor activity. In many instances, movement and muscle artifact can dominate the EEG, rendering its analysis impossible. In such instances, analysis of the video component becomes the predominant basis for diagnosis. That could be potentially misleading, as epileptic seizures can be very bizarre in their manifestations, with minimal associated EEG change when they arise from the mesial frontal or orbitofrontal region.

The video analysis of psychogenic seizures should also take into consideration that no single feature or even combination of features are totally specific. It is not uncommon for rhythmic movement to be associated with rhythmic motion artifact that could mislead into a diagnosis of seizure activity. Clues to the diagnosis could come from brief quiet periods that still include unresponsiveness or from the immediate postictal state when the patient is still unresponsive but quiet, allowing for a perfectly normal EEG to show through. When such periods are absent, the pattern of artifact can be helpful.

The rhythmic activity frequency, morphology and amplitude will usually evolve, or at least fluctuate in epileptic seizures. The rhythmic activity associated with non-epileptic seizures is either constant in its frequency or includes irregularities that reflect on the EEG artifact. Since psychogenic seizures are at times discontinuous, the associated artifact can also be discontinuous.

The occurrence of seizures immediately out of sleep is strong evidence against nonepileptic psychogenic seizure diagnosis. However, some patients with psychogenic seizures report that attacks occur out of sleep, but the EEG will usually demonstrate a waking background at onset.

Testing patients during events

In epilepsy monitoring units where patients are observed continuously and in any short-term video-EEG monitoring where an EEG technologist is present, the testing of patients during events is of great clinical utility.

Testing is aimed at the following:

- Establish if the patient is unresponsive
- Determine if there is impairment in specific areas
- Determine if the patient has recollection for items given during the spell, or for events that occurred during the spell

The authors suggest that the patient's ability to follow commands and to name items be tested at baseline. Should a suspicious ictal EEG activity appear or any behavioral changes occur that are suggestive of a seizure, then the patient should be given a command, the response to which can be assessed visually upon video review. For example, the patient could be asked to point to the ceiling, touch his/her nose, or clap the hands. The patient can then be given items to name and to remember. One study used a sentence from the Boston Diagnostic Aphasic Battery, "I heard him speak on the radio last night," to assess reading abilities postictally.

Patients with left temporal seizures usually required more than one minute to read the sentence correctly from the termination of the seizure. Patients with right temporal lobe seizures were able to read the sentence within one minute from seizure termination. When the patient has fully recovered, memory can be tested by asking for items given during the seizure as well as for events during a seizure. For example, it is not uncommon for patients with right temporal lobe seizures to produce spontaneous sentences (often with a tinge of fear) and respond almost normally to commands or other verbal stimuli. Once the seizure is over, it is quite common for these patients not to remember the conversation.

Testing during discharges precipitated by hyperventilation

Testing is sometimes useful to identify whether a seizure has occurred or the EEG discharge was subclinical/asymptomatic. In patients with generalized absence seizures, it is recognized that even a single spike-and-wave discharge is usually associated with a change when sufficiently sensitive testing is used. However, the degree of alteration of responsiveness and awareness varies tremendously between patients such that some patients have no gross detectable change. Such determination can be very useful in order to recommend restrictions on activity. As a result of the above, testing patients' responsiveness during generalized spike-and-wave discharges should be routine when the EEG technologist is present during the baseline EEG or a session of short-term monitoring.

During hyperventilation, a common EEG response is generalized bisynchronous delta activity that is totally within normal, particularly for younger children. However, a rare pattern of absence seizures involve 3 Hz delta activity without concomitant spikes (as shown on the disc). Because of this pattern, it is also advisable to test patients who have a sustained generalized 3 Hz delta activity during hyperventilation, to determine if responsiveness is altered. A definite diagnosis of absence seizures is not possible without demonstrating a clinical alteration.

Chapter 9.
Seizure Semiology and Differential Diagnosis

The authors chose to adhere mainly to the older and more widely used classification schemes rather than the less widely used yet thoughtful schemes that are in development. However, we have incorporated the terminology of some seizure types that were not listed in older classifications. Future editions of this work will reflect new schemes when fully established.

Seizure classification

The international classification of seizures divides seizures into two major groups, *partial* (or focal or local) and *generalized*. The subdivision is dependent on whether the onset is in one part of one hemisphere or in both hemispheres simultaneously. Partial seizures are further subdivided into simple partial, complex partial, and partial becoming secondarily generalized. Simple partial seizures do not affect awareness or responsiveness, whereas complex partial seizures are associated with impairment or complete loss of awareness or responsiveness. Partial seizures vary remarkably in their manifestations, depending on where they originate, where they spread and how fast they spread. Generalized seizure types include absence (typical or atypical), myoclonic, clonic, tonic, tonic-clonic, and atonic seizures. Generalized seizure types are more homogeneous in their clinical manifestations, though they have a wide spectrum of severity. Partial seizure semiology will be discussed first, based on the lobe of origin. The classification below includes components outside the last international classification of epileptic seizures.

Partial seizure types

Initial symptoms of partial seizures depend to a large extent on the site of origin of the discharge. Partial seizures may originate in any lobe. However, complex partial seizures most commonly have a temporal lobe focus. The classification of seizure manifestations by site of origin is not part of the international seizure classification, but is extremely useful. The most common localizations of site of partial seizure onset, are in order:

- Temporal
- Frontal
- Parietal
- Occipital

Seizures may also arise in the insular lobe. Origin in subcortical structures and the cerebellum is extremely rare and will not be addressed. Partial seizures originating in any of the lobes can be simple partial, complex partial or secondarily generalized depending on the spread of seizure activity.

Temporal

Temporal lobe epilepsy (TLE) is the most common symptomatic/ cryptogenic partial epilepsy. The characteristic manifestations of temporal lobe seizures have long been recognized. However, the advent of EEG-video monitoring and its use in presurgical evaluation have had a great impact on the understanding of temporal lobe seizure semiology. Temporal lobe epilepsy is often refractory to medical therapy, and is often amenable to surgical treatment. The surgical outcome is dependent on accurate localization of the epileptogenic focus. The analysis of clinical semiology in patients who were seizure-free after temporal lobectomy versus those still experiencing seizures has helped identify manifestations characteristic of temporal lobe origin, and those that suggest extratemporal localization. In addition, specific seizure manifestations were analyzed for their lateralizing value and their localizing value within the temporal lobe.

Seizure aura

Most patients with TLE report a seizure aura. This is particularly true in mesial TLE, by far the largest TLE group. In a selected patient group with proven mesial temporal lobe origin, more than 90% of patients reported an aura. The most common was an epigastric aura. Although no aura is totally specific for temporal lobe seizures, some are very strongly associated with a temporal lobe origin, particularly viscerosensory (such as epigastric sensation) and experiential or psychic auras (such as "deja-vu"). Both of these types of aura are more likely with right temporal foci, but this is only a trend. Whereas viscerosensory auras are generally more common in mesial TLE associated with hippocampal sclerosis, experiential auras and deja vu in particular are more common in the benign familial temporal lobe epilepsy syndrome. Chills and goosebumps are more common with left temporal foci, and if they are unilateral, they are usually ipsilateral to the seizure focus. An auditory aura is very suggestive of lateral temporal origin. This can be a positive (for example, ringing sound) or negative symptom (loss of hearing). The auditory aura is a hallmark of an autosomal dominant form of lateral temporal lobe epilepsy. Cephalic auras (nonspecific sensation in the head) and vertigo are more likely extratemporal. The same is true of somatosensory and visual auras. Absence of an aura is more likely with bitemporal than unilateral temporal epilepsy.

Motor manifestations

The complex partial phase of mesial temporal lobe seizures usually starts with motor arrest or motionless staring, oroalimentary automatisms, or non-specific extremity automatisms.

Oroalimentary automatisms, mainly lip smacking, chewing and swallowing movements are suggestive of temporal lobe involvement. However, they may reflect spread of seizure activity to the temporal lobe from other locations, and can also be seen in a more subtle form in absence seizures, or postictally in a variety of seizure types.

Spitting and drinking automatisms suggest right temporal localization.

Automatisms with preserved responsiveness also favor right temporal localization.

Extremity automatisms are less specific and can be seen in temporal as well as extratemporal epilepsy. However, the progression of these automatisms is more gradual in temporal lobe epilepsy. In extratemporal epilepsy, they tend to have an abrupt bilateral onset and a frenzied character. Automatisms in themselves have no lateralizing value. However, the extremity contralateral to the side of the focus is often involved in dystonic posturing or immobility and may therefore not demonstrate automatisms. In this instance, automatisms will predominate in the extremity ipsilateral to the seizure focus. This may lead to confusion for the inexperienced observer who may interpret repetitive automatisms as clonic activity.

Defined in the strictest manner, *dystonic posturing* is an unnatural position that includes a rotatory component. Dystonic posturing has been associated with ictal activation in the contralateral putamen. There is evidence that there is a spectrum of posturing, with classical dystonic posturing at one extreme, and simple immobility of an extremity at the other, including subtle posturing without a clear demonstrated rotatory component in between. Dystonic posturing has a strong lateralizing value in temporal lobe epilepsy. However, as with any other manifestations, late occurrence could represent activation of the contralateral side and may therefore have a lesser value.

Head turning in temporal lobe epilepsy has been the subject of great controversy. Current evidence suggests that early head turning, particularly that associated with dystonic posturing, tends to be ipsilateral to the focus. Its mechanism is not well defined. Some have suggested it could represent neglect of the contralateral hemisphere. However, in many instances the early head turning is of a tonic nature, which raises the possibility of a motor drive, possibly from the basal ganglia. In one study, the occurrence of head turning within 30 seconds of seizure onset, in association with dystonic posturing, and not leading to secondarily generalization was strictly ipsilateral to the temporal seizure focus. Late head turning, on the other hand, is more likely to be contralateral. Head turning that leads to secondary generalization can have a tonic or clonic character and has been termed "versive" or "adversive." Versive head turning is almost always contralateral to the seizure focus. However, an ipsilateral versive head turn has been noted towards the end of secondarily generalized tonic-clonic seizures in some patients.

Language manifestations

Language manifestations are potentially very valuable in lateralizing temporal lobe seizure origin.

Ictal speech arrest does not seem to have lateralizing value. It may be due to disruption of language mechanisms, to loss of awareness/responsiveness, or to a positive or negative motor effect. There is a suggestion, however, that in temporal simple partial seizures a speech arrest could represent aphasia and may thus be lateralizing to the dominant temporal lobe.

Well-formed ictal language strongly suggests a non-dominant right temporal lobe focus. This is not true, however, of single words or non-verbal vocalizations. Ictal vocalization has limited specificity with respect to localization or lateralization. The well-formed ictal language in some patients with right temporal lobe seizures has a tinge of fear. For example, it is not uncommon for patients to utter "I'm sick, I'm sick" or "I'm going to die, don't let me die." In most instances, however, the patient does not remember these utterances, and fear may not be a known component of the semiology.

Ictal jargon is rare but has been associated with dominant temporal lobe foci. It may reflect a partial disruption of language mechanisms as seen in chronic Wernicke's aphasia.

Global aphasia may occur in association with localized simple partial seizures restricted in the temporal lobe, including the basal temporal language area. Chronic temporal lobe lesions do not produce global aphasia. However, acute electrical stimulation in Wernicke's area as well as basal temporal language area does produce global aphasia, perhaps because compensatory mechanisms have not had the chance to be activated. Global aphasia in simple partial seizures therefore could be consistent with a left dominant temporal localization.

Postictal aphasia is strongly associated with a left dominant temporal localization. In patients with atypical language representation, the lateralizing significance of language dysfunction has to be reinterpreted. In one study, all patients with right temporal seizures were able to correctly read a test sentence within one minute of seizure termination while patients with dominant left temporal foci had disruption of reading for more than one minute.

Other signs

A variety of other manifestations may have lateralizing value.

Ictal vomiting has been associated with right-sided foci. However, this is not uniform, and vomiting may also be a manifestation of extratemporal foci.

Unilateral eye blinking tends to be ipsilateral to seizure origin.

Focal facial motor activity early in the seizure favors a lateral neocortical origin, usually contralateral to the side of jerking.

Transition to secondary generalization

The motor manifestations during transition to secondary generalization can be very valuable in lateralization. Versive head turning, tonic posturing, and clonic activity are most often contralateral to seizure origin. Occasionally, however, they can be falsely lateralizing if there is contralateral seizure spread prior to generalization.

Postictal manifestations

- *Postictal cough* has been found predominately following right temporal seizures
- *Postictal nose wiping* tends to be performed with the hand ipsilateral to the seizure focus
- *Postictal urinary urgency* suggests a right temporal localization

None of the above signs is significant in isolation. However, the combination of several signs and symptoms can be a powerful tool in localizing and lateralizing temporal lobe epilepsy. The addition of semiological information unquestionably enhances the localizing ability of the presurgical evaluation.

Frontal

Aura

The frontal lobe is the second most common source of seizures after the temporal lobe. A great variety of seizure manifestations can be related to frontal lobe origin. An aura is less common with frontal than with temporal lobe origin. There is also only a limited specificity in auras. For example, autonomic auras with abdominal sensation are more likely to be of temporal lobe origin. However, frontal lobe limbic seizures may have the same autonomic auras, including epigastric sensation. These autonomic auras have been ascribed to the orbitofrontal and the cingulate regions. Somatosensory auras are generally ascribed to activation of the primary sensory cortex. However, frontal lobe seizures originating in the supplementary motor area are frequently associated with a sensory aura due to activation of the supplementary sensory area. The sensory auras related to supplementary motor seizures generally do not have a march, are more often proximal, and may be bilateral in distribution although a contralateral occurrence is most likely. Perhaps the most common aura in frontal lobe seizures is the non-specific cephalic sensation, which has no localizing value. It has been suggested that isolated auras are a common feature of temporal lobe but not frontal lobe epilepsy. Thus, many patients with frontal lobe epilepsy deny auras that do not progress further.

Motor manifestations

Activation of the primary motor cortex is well known to be associated with clonic activity. Focal clonic or tonic-clonic seizures therefore are most likely originating in the primary motor cortex. "Focal cortical myoclonus" is another manifestation of primary motor cortex epileptogenicity. In general, consciousness may be completely preserved unless there has been spread of seizure activity to the contralateral hemisphere.

Supplementary motor seizures also tend to be simple partial seizures, with no alteration of consciousness. They are characterized by posturing that can affect one limb, two limbs, or all four extremities. This is a notable exception to the rule that bilateral seizure activity should be accompanied by loss of consciousness. These seizures tend to be brief in duration, tend to cluster, and tend to be predominately nocturnal and sleep related. Since the seizure origin is in mesial frontal cortex, there is often no recorded interictal or ictal EEG activity due to the unfavorable dipole orientation. These seizures are frequently misdiagnosed as psychogenic due to the above features. Withdrawal of antiepileptic drug therapy may be associated with evolution to secondary generalized tonic-clonic seizure activity, which is easily recognized, and results in eventual correct diagnosis. The posturing of the extremities is predominately proximal while the hands and fingers or feet and toes seem to be free and patients will frequently wiggle the distal extremities. There is often a vocalization of moaning or groaning and the patient reports being unable to breathe.

Bizarre complex partial seizures have been ascribed to seizure origin in the cingulate gyrus or orbitofrontal region. Such seizures are frequently characterized by frenetic gestural automatisms that are often bilateral, unless there is associated contralateral posturing. These automatisms can be bizarre and can be associated with bizarre vocalizations and verbalizations, including expletives. These seizures tend to be short and associated with only brief postictal manifestations. Again, the clinical features and the frequent absence of interictal epileptiform activity as well as absence or masking of ictal EEG manifestations have frequently resulted in the diagnosis of psychogenic seizures.

Seizures originating in the anterior-mesial frontal region at times imitate absence seizures through rapid secondary bilateral synchrony. These seizures are frequently referred to as *frontal absences*. They can clinically be characterized by altered responsiveness and arrest of activity for a few seconds with rapid return to baseline, and minimal postictal manifestations. Such seizures can be totally indistinguishable from generalized absence seizures, except for the presence of a frontal lesion, and at times the presence of consistent asymmetry on EEG. Seizures of frontal lobe origin seizures can imitate a variety of other generalized seizure types, including generalized tonic, generalized atonic and generalized tonic-clonic seizures. Frontal lobe seizures are recognized to have a more rapid spread to the contralateral hemisphere. This is partly why falling (drop attacks) and incontinence seem more likely with frontal lobe seizures.

The lateralizing value of signs in frontal lobe seizures may be less than with temporal lobe seizures, due to the propensity for rapid contralateral spread and contralateral hemisphere activation.

Parietal

The parietal lobe is the next most likely source of seizures after temporal and frontal lobe. The best recognized manifestation of parietal lobe origin is a sensory aura, particularly if there is an associated march. The sensation can be described as numbness, tingling, pins and needles, burning, or can be a nondescript one.

Sensory march is strongly suggestive of a post central, primary sensory cortex involvement.

Sensory aura without march can originate in the second sensory area, which is located over the parietal operculum. Although the manifestations there are most often contralateral, they are occasionally ipsilateral or bilateral.

Vertigo, difficulty localizing body position in space, sensation that a body part is moving, or that an extremity is absent are other less common sensory auras that suggest a parietal lobe origin.

Focal weakness has also been described with parietal foci. Such seizures have been referred to as focal inhibitory motor seizures or focal atonic seizures. They frequently have a preceding sensory aura.

Seizures without parietal lobe symptoms. Most patients with parietal lobe epilepsy have no parietal lobe symptoms but rather manifestations resulting from spread to occipital, temporal, or frontal lobe.

Common manifestations include:

- Contralateral tonic posturing
- Focal clonic activity
- Generalized asymmetrical tonic posturing
- Head and eye deviation, described in almost 50% of patients

When complex partial seizures occur, they can be characterized by:

- Staring
- Relative immobility with minimal automatisms

or

- Hyperkinetic motor activity (uncommonly)

Occipital

Sensory symptoms suggesting occipital origin are:

- *Visual aura* is the key manifestation that suggests occipital lobe origin.
- *Elementary visual hallucinations* strongly suggest involvement of primary visual cortex. These hallucinations may be black or white or colored. They can be flashing or steady. They can be stationary or moving. There may be distortion of vision, and there may also be a loss of vision. The *ictal blindness* can be a blackout or a whiteout. If this is in one field, it strongly suggests seizure activity contralateral to that field. More complex visual hallucinations such as ones involving scenes suggest involvement of the occiptotemporal junction.
- *Auditory hallucinations, vertigo, focal sensory experiences* may also be seen, but suggest seizure spread to the lateral temporal or parietal regions.

Motor symptoms suggesting occipital origin include:

- Bilateral blinking
- Eye deviation, usually contralateral

One distinctive feature of occipital lobe seizures that develop and propagate posteriorly is the slow progression of ictal manifestations. For example, the eye deviation that is seen with occipital lobe origin tends to be a lot slower than that noted with frontal lobe origin.

Insular

Insular seizures are not well characterized. It is thought that activation of the insula may be responsible for the abdominal sensation that is so common in mesial temporal lobe epilepsy.

Other seizure manifestations considered possibly related to the insula include hyperventilation and hypersalivation. Seizures originating in the insula often involve an initial constricting laryngeal sensation, paresthesias over the face or a wide area of the body contralateral to the focus, then dysarthric speech, then focal tonic or clonic activity.

Select features that may suggest lobe localization					
Lobe of onset	Mesial temporal	Lateral temporal	Frontal	Parietal	Occipital
Aura	Epigastric sensation; deja-vu	Auditory experience	None-cephalic aura (not specific)	Sensory aura with march	Elementary visual hallucination
Motor manifestations	Oroalimentary automatism, Gradual development of simple extremity automatisms Dystonic posturing-contralateral	Early facial twitching	Abrupt posturing, bizarre gestural automatisms	Variable	Blinking, nystagmus
Head turning	Early ipsilateral, nonversive	Variable	fast contralateral versive head turning	Variable	Slow contralateral versive head turn
Verbalization-vocalization	Well formed sentences if right (nondominant) temporal	Rhythmic vocalization with facial twitching	May have complex vocalizations including expletives	Variable	Variable- may describe visual hallucinations in nondominant
Generalization	Infrequent	Frequent	Frequent	Variable	Variable
Seizure duration	Long (2-3 minutes)	Generally shorter	Short (30 sec-1 min)	Variable	Variable
Postictal state	Can be prolonged with postictal aphasia if dominant temporal		Short	Variable	Variable

Generalized seizure types

Generalized seizures are divided into multiple types. What is in common between generalized seizure types is bilateral onset clinically and by EEG. However, the circuits involved in different seizure types are likely to be very different.

Generalized absence seizures

These seizures can occur in a variety of epileptic syndromes, particularly childhood absence epilepsy and juvenile absence epilepsy. These seizures are characterized by sudden onset without any aura, brief duration, typically less than 15 seconds, and sudden termination without any postictal state. Typically, there is suspension of awareness and arrest of activity during the episodes, but some subtle motor manifestations are quite common.

Simple automatisms are most common, particularly perseverative automatisms. Automatisms may include fumbling with an object that the patient was holding, rubbing a body part, or licking the lips. Automatisms are more likely with longer duration of absence seizure activity.

Myoclonus is the next most common motor manifestation. This includes blinking and subtle twitching of the fingers.

Tonic features may occur with uprolling of the eyes and slight stiffening of the neck with neck extension, though this is mild.

Atonic components can also be seen, with slight decrease of tone and slumping, again to a mild degree.

Autonomic manifestations may occur, including pupillary dilation, piloerection, and infrequently, incontinence.

At times, consciousness is partially preserved during absence seizures. This is more likely to occur in adults who have had persistent absence seizures from childhood. When there is some preservation of awareness but loss of responsiveness, patients may describe some subjective experiences that could erroneously suggest an aura. For example, lightheadedness or spaciness may be reported. In addition, some patients report "confusion" after the seizure. This usually reflects the effect of missing parts of a conversation rather than true confusion.

Atypical absence seizures.

This variant of generalized absence seizures tends to occur in symptomatic generalized epilepsy such as Lennox-Gastaut syndrome. The main distinction between typical and atypical absence seizures is electrographic, as the latter have a slower frequency of less than 2.5 Hz. Clinical distinctive features reported are a slower loss of awareness and a more gradual recovery, as well as perhaps more prominent motor manifestations.

Generalized absence seizures with eyelid myoclonia

These seizures occur predominately in women, as part of an epileptic syndrome. In this syndrome, eyelid myoclonia may occur with or without associated spike-and-wave activity.

Myoclonic absences

These seizures associated with the typical 2.5 to 3.5 Hz spike-and-wave discharge differ from absence seizures by the presence of a very prominent clonic activity at the same frequency as the spike-and-wave discharges. The seizures in this syndrome tend to be harder to control.

Generalized myoclonic seizures

Generalized myoclonic seizures last a fraction of a second. They vary in severity from mild with barely visible twitch to severe with massive myoclonus associated with falling. The myoclonic jerk may involve the whole body, or the upper extremities or the head alone. Although they are usually bilateral, they could be unilateral with shifting lateralization. Myoclonic seizures are not associated with loss of consciousness because of their very brief duration. They often occur in clusters and patients occasionally report some disruption of consciousness with a cluster of closely spaced seizures.

Generalized myoclonic seizures are to be distinguished from non-epileptic myoclonus, which can originate at any level of the central nervous system.

Generalized clonic seizures

These seizures are characterized by rhythmic bilateral clonic jerking starting with loss of consciousness. They are infrequent.

Generalized tonic seizures

These seizures occur most often in neurologically impaired individuals. They are characterized by sudden loss of consciousness with generalized tonic posturing that may be asymmetrical. These seizures can be difficult to distinguish from partial onset seizures of frontal or parietal origin. The posturing/stiffening can be generalized and massive or minimal, manifesting only with eye opening or with slight neck extension.

Tonic seizures can be abrupt or can manifest with slow posturing. They are more likely to occur out of sleep. They are typically quite brief but may have a postictal state with a duration and severity that are disproportionate to the seizure duration.

The most common pattern of generalized tonic seizure posturing involves flexion of the trunk and extension of the extremities with abduction at the shoulders. There may be associated vocalization, particularly with the massive and abrupt generalized tonic seizures.

Generalized atonic seizures

These seizures can vary in manifestation from subtle drooping of the head to a massive loss of tone with falling. They are more common in children. They are associated with drop attacks. However, drop attacks can be due to tonic seizures as well, and the distinction of the two can be difficult without direct observation.

Generalized myoclonic-atonic seizures

These seizures are commonly part of the syndrome of myoclonic astatic epilepsy, also referred to as Doose's syndrome. In these seizures, a myoclonic jerk precedes the loss of tone. The seizures are very brief with rapid recovery. However, injuries are not uncommon, due to falls from loss of tone.

Generalized negative epileptic myoclonus

Negative epileptic myoclonus is similar to epileptic myoclonic seizures, but is associated with very brief loss of tone that may not be appreciated unless the affected extremities are elevated or engaged in other activity. An analogy can be made with asterixis, which resembles non-epileptic myoclonus, but with momentary loss of tone rather than momentary contraction,

Pseudoseizures (nonepileptic psychogenic seizures)

Clinical presentations

A major role of EEG monitoring units is differentiation of epileptic seizures from pseudoseizures. The spectrum of clinical presentations of pseudoseizures is almost as broad as that of epileptic seizures. There is no single clinical pattern of non-epileptic psychogenic seizures. Most commonly, these include some motor activity. One clinical classification of psychogenic seizures includes the following categories:

- Generalized convulsive activity, somewhat imitating generalized tonic-clonic seizures
- Focal, lateralized, or migratory motor activity
- Collapse
- Altered responsiveness without any motor activity

All studies analyzing clinical features of psychogenic seizures and comparing them to epileptic seizures indicate clearly that no single feature is definitive. When comparing psychogenic seizures with generalized motor activity and true generalized tonic-clonic seizures, features that helped discriminate the two were

- out of phase upper extremity movements
- out of phase lower extremity movements
- absence of vocalization, or initiation of the seizure with vocalization
- forward pelvic thrusting
- absence of body rigidity during generalized jerking

Combining two or more of the above features provided more than 90% accuracy in discrimination between epileptic generalized tonic-clonic seizures and psychogenic events with generalized motor activity. However, when these features were considered to distinguish psychogenic seizures from frontal lobe complex partial seizures, they lost their discriminative value (see below).

The pattern of involvement of facial muscles during the event is also very useful. Sustained forceful eye closure with active resistance to eye opening is common with psychogenic seizures. Similarly, the presence of a clenched mouth during a motor seizure is atypical for epilepsy.

Biting of the lip or tip of the tongue is also atypical for epileptic attacks. Epileptic seizures are usually associated with biting injury on the side of the tongue.

Other features that suggest a psychogenic origin include

- precipitation by suggestion
- gradual onset
- pre-ictal behavioral changes (typically intermittent, resembling preparation for the full-fledged motor event)
- pseudo-sleep before seizure onset
- discontinuous motor activity

- prolonged duration (pseudo status epilepticus is common)
- gradual cessation
- absence of postictal state (but this is common with bizarre frontal lobe complex partial seizures)
- high seizure frequency
- excessive variability in ictal manifestations
- non-physiologic progression
- eye fluttering
- vocalizations consisting of gagging, retching, gasping, screaming, crying or moaning
- retained consciousness and recollection of events with bilateral jerking activity (however this may also occur with generalized myoclonic and supplementary motor seizures)
- precipitation of typical attacks by suggestion, and termination of a prolonged event with suggestion
- emotional display during events, such as weeping
- the occurrence of events only in the presence of others

Incontinence during a seizure is suggestive of an epileptic origin, but may be seen with non-epileptic seizures, particularly if there is an underlying depressive psychopathology. Self-injury is unlikely to present itself in the epilepsy monitoring unit. This is more common in patients with true epilepsy, but can certainly occur in non-epileptic seizures with an underlying depression.

As mentioned above, frontal lobe complex partial seizures can be bizarre and difficult to distinguish from pseudoseizures. Frontal lobe complex partial seizures and non-epileptic psychogenic seizures do not differ from each other with respect to pelvic thrusting, rocking of body, or side-to-side head movements. The features that favor frontal lobe partial seizures are:

- turning to a prone position during a seizure- occurred only in frontal lobe partial seizures.
- nocturnal occurrence
- short ictal duration
- stereotyped pattern of movements

Another seizure type that may be confused with pseudoseizures is supplementary motor seizures. These involve posturing of extremities (could be all four), usually with preserved consciousness. Supplementary motor seizures were distinguished from psychogenic seizures by

- short duration
- stereotyped pattern
- tendency to occur in sleep
- typical tonic contraction of the upper extremities in abduction

Thus, if seizures with side-to-side head motion and forward pelvic thrusting also had a prolonged duration, pseudoseizures would be most likely.

Appendix: Readings

The information contained in this work is distilled from thousands of scientific papers and many years of clinical practice. In this concise text, it was impossible to list all of these valuable works. A brief list of important works which should be in the library of the neurophysiologist is as follows.

Books

EEG

Fisch BJ. Fisch and Spehlmann's EEG Primer, 3rd Edition. Elsevier, 1999.

Hughes, JR. EEG in Clinical Practice, 2nd edition. Butterworth-Heinemann, 1994.

Ebersole JS, Pedley TA (Eds). Current Practice of Clinical Electroencephalography, 3rd Edition. Lippincott Williams & Wilkins, 2003

Misulis KE, Head TC; Essentials of Clinical Neurophysiology, 3rd edition. Butterworth-Heinemann, 2003.

Niedermeyer E, Lopes Da Silva F (Eds). Electroencephalography: Basic Principles, Clinical Applications, and Related Fields. Lippincott Williams & Wilkins, 1999.

Blume WT, Kaibara M. Atlas of Adult Electroencephalography. Raven Press, 1995.

Blume WT, Kaibara M. Atlas of Pediatric Electroencephalography, 2nd edition. Lippincott Raven, 1999.

Epilepsy

Engel, J. Jr. and Pedley, T.A. (Eds). Epilepsy: A Comprehensive Textbook. Vols. 1, 2 and 3. Lippincott-Raven, 1997.

Wyllie E. (Ed). The Treatment of Epilepsy: Principles and Practice, 3rd edition. Elaine Wyllie. Lippincott Williams & Wilkins, 2001.

Lüders HO, Noachtar S. Atlas of Epileptic Seizures and Syndromes. WB Saunders, 2001.

Lüders HO, Noachtar S. Atlas and Classification of Electroencephalography. WB Saunders, 1999.

Roger J, Dravet C, Bureau M, Dreifuss FE, Wolf P. Epileptic Syndromes in Infancy, Childhood and Adolescence. John Libbey 1985.

Papers

Classification

Commission on Classification and Terminology of the International League Against Epilepsy. Proposal for revised clinical and electroencephalographic classification of epileptic seizures. Epilepsia 1981;22:489-501.

Commission on Classification and Terminology of the International League Against Epilepsy. Proposal for classification of epilepsies and epileptic syndromes. Epilepsia 1985;26:268-78.

Luders H, Acharya J, Baumgartner C, Benbadis S, Bleasel A, Burgess R, Dinner DS, Ebner A, Foldvary N, Geller E, Hamer H, Holthausen H, Kotagal P, Morris H, Meencke HJ, Noachtar S, Rosenow F, Sakamoto A, Steinhoff BJ, Tuxhorn I, Wyllie E. Semiological seizure classification. Epilepsia 1998;39:1006-13.

Engel J Jr. A proposed diagnostic scheme for people with epileptic seizures and with epilepsy: report of the ILAE Task Force on Classification and Terminology. Epilepsia 2001;42:796-803.

Seizure Semiology

Auras

Palmini A, Gloor P. The localizing value of auras in partial seizures: a prospective and retrospective study. Neurology 1992;42:801-8.

Mesial Temporal lobe seizures

Kotagal P, Luders H, Morris HH, Dinner DS, Wyllie E, Godoy J, Rothner AD. Dystonic posturing in complex partial seizures of temporal lobe onset: a new lateralizing sign. Neurology 1989;39:196-201.

Chee MW, Kotagal P, Van Ness PC, Gragg L, Murphy D, Luders HO. Lateralizing signs in intractable partial epilepsy: blinded multiple-observer analysis. Neurology 1993;43:2519-25.

Gabr M, Luders H, Dinner D, Morris H, Wyllie E. Speech manifestations in lateralization of temporal lobe seizures. Ann Neurol 1989;25:82-7.

Privitera MD, Morris GL, Gilliam F. Postictal language assessment and lateralization of complex partial seizures. Ann Neurol 1991;30:391-6.

Fakhoury T, Abou-Khalil B, Peguero E. Differentiating clinical features of right and left temporal lobe seizures. Epilepsia 1994;35:1038-44.

Fakhoury T, Abou-Khalil B. Association of ipsilateral head turning and dystonia in temporal lobe seizures. Epilepsia 1995;36:1065-70.

Williamson PD, Thadani VM, French JA, Darcey TM, Mattson RH, Spencer SS, Spencer DD. Medial temporal lobe epilepsy: videotape analysis of objective clinical seizure characteristics. Epilepsia 1998;39:1182-8.

Foldvary N, Lee N, Thwaites G, Mascha E, Hammel J, Kim H, Friedman AH, Radtke RA. Clinical and electrographic manifestations of lesional neocortical temporal lobe epilepsy. Neurology 1997;49:757-63.

Maillard L, Vignal JP, Gavaret M, Guye M, Biraben A, McGonigal A, Chauvel P, Bartolomei F. Semiologic and electrophysiologic correlations in temporal lobe seizure subtypes. Epilepsia 2004;45:1590-9.

Gil-Nagel A, Risinger MW. Ictal semiology in hippocampal versus extrahippocampal temporal lobe epilepsy. Brain 1997;120:183-92.

Dupont S, Semah F, Boon P, Saint-Hilaire JM, Adam C, Broglin D, Baulac M. Association of ipsilateral motor automatisms and contralateral dystonic posturing: a clinical feature differentiating medial from neocortical temporal lobe epilepsy. Arch Neurol 1999;56:927-32.

Frontal lobe seizures

Williamson PD, Spencer DD, Spencer SS, Novelly RA, Mattson RH. Complex partial seizures of frontal lobe origin. Ann Neurol 1985;18:497-504.

Salanova V, Morris HH, Van Ness P, Kotagal P, Wyllie E, Luders H. Frontal lobe seizures: electroclinical syndromes. Epilepsia 1995;36:16-24.

Morris HH 3rd, Dinner DS, Luders H, Wyllie E, Kramer R. Supplementary motor seizures: clinical and electroencephalographic findings. Neurology 1988;38:1075-82.

Occipital Lobe seizures

Williamson PD, Thadani VM, Darcey TM, Spencer DD, Spencer SS, Mattson RH. Occipital lobe epilepsy: clinical characteristics, seizure spread patterns, and results of surgery. Ann Neurol 1992;31:3-13.

Salanova V, Andermann F, Olivier A, Rasmussen T, Quesney LF. Occipital lobe epilepsy: electroclinical manifestations, electrocorticography, cortical stimulation and outcome in 42 patients treated between 1930 and 1991. Surgery of occipital lobe epilepsy. Brain 1992;115:1655-80.

Parietal lobe seizures

Williamson PD, Boon PA, Thadani VM, Darcey TM, Spencer DD, Spencer SS, Novelly RA, Mattson RH. Parietal lobe epilepsy: diagnostic considerations and results of surgery. Ann Neurol 1992;31:193-201.

Salanova V, Andermann F, Rasmussen T, Olivier A, Quesney LF. Parietal lobe epilepsy. Clinical manifestations and outcome in 82 patients treated surgically between 1929 and 1988. Brain 1995;118:607-27.

Insular seizures

Isnard J, Guenot M, Sindou M, Mauguiere F. Clinical manifestations of insular lobe seizures: a stereo-electroencephalographic study. Epilepsia 2004;45:1079-90.

Secondarily generalized seizures

Wyllie E, Luders H, Morris HH, Lesser RP, Dinner DS. The lateralizing significance of versive head and eye movements during epileptic seizures. Neurology 1986;36:606-11.

Theodore WH, Porter RJ, Albert P, Kelley K, Bromfield E, Devinsky O, Sato S. The secondarily generalized tonic-clonic seizure: a videotape analysis. Neurology 1994;44:1403-7.

Niaz FE, Abou-Khalil B, Fakhoury T. The generalized tonic-clonic seizure in partial versus generalized epilepsy: semiologic differences. Epilepsia 1999;40:1664-6.

Jobst BC, Williamson PD, Neuschwander TB, Darcey TM, Thadani VM, Roberts DW. Secondarily generalized seizures in mesial temporal epilepsy: clinical characteristics, lateralizing signs, and association with sleep-wake cycle. Epilepsia 2001;42:1279-87.

Pseudoseizures

Gulick TA, Spinks IP, King DW. Pseudoseizures: ictal phenomena. Neurology 1982;32:24-30.

Gates JR, Ramani V, Whalen S, Loewenson R. Ictal characteristics of pseudoseizures. Arch Neurol 1985;42:1183-7.

Kanner AM, Morris HH, Luders H, Dinner DS, Wyllie E, Medendorp SV, Rowan AJ. Supplementary motor seizures mimicking pseudoseizures: some clinical differences. Neurology 1990;40:1404-7.

Saygi S, Katz A, Marks DA, Spencer SS. Frontal lobe partial seizures and psychogenic seizures: comparison of clinical and ictal characteristics. Neurology 1992;42:1274-7.

Lesser RP. Psychogenic seizures. Neurology 1996;46:1499-507

DeToledo JC, Ramsay RE. Patterns of involvement of facial muscles during epileptic and nonepileptic events: review of 654 events. Neurology 1996;47:621-5.

Benbadis SR, Lancman ME, King LM, Swanson SJ. Preictal pseudosleep: a new finding in psychogenic seizures. Neurology 1996;47:63-7.

Ictal EEG

Risinger MW, Engel J Jr, Van Ness PC, Henry TR, Crandall PH. Ictal localization of temporal lobe seizures with scalp/sphenoidal recordings. Neurology 1989;39:1288-93.

Ebersole JS, Pacia SV. Localization of temporal lobe foci by ictal EEG patterns. Epilepsia 1996;37:386-99.

Foldvary N, Klem G, Hammel J, Bingaman W, Najm I, Luders H. The localizing value of ictal EEG in focal epilepsy. Neurology 2001;57:2022-8.

Bautista RE, Spencer DD, Spencer SS. EEG findings in frontal lobe epilepsies. Neurology 1998;50:1765-71.

Worrell GA, So EL, Kazemi J, O'Brien TJ, Mosewich RK, Cascino GD, Meyer FB, Marsh WR. Focal ictal beta discharge on scalp EEG predicts excellent outcome of frontal lobe epilepsy surgery. Epilepsia 2002;43:277-82.

Internet sites

- Epilepsy Foundation: www.efa.org
- International League Against Epilepsy: www.ilae-epilepsy.org
- The epilepsy project: www.epilepsy.com
- American epilepsy society: www.aesnet.org